THE
MALE
CLIMACTERIC

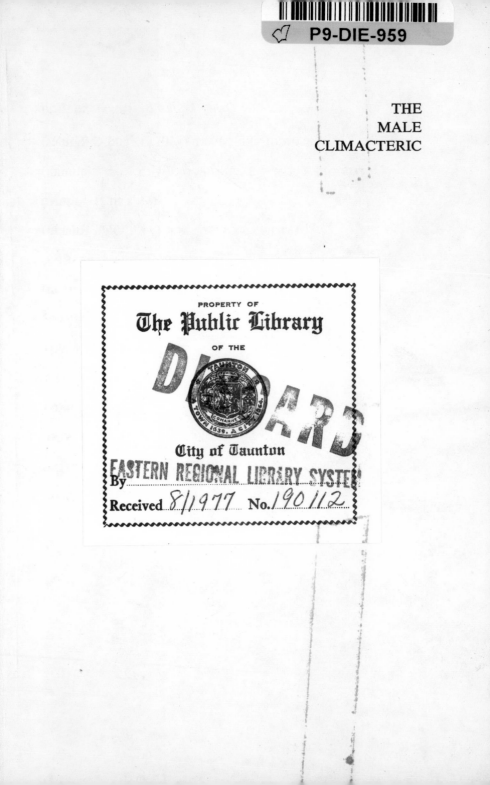

The Male Climacteric

Helmut J. Ruebsaat, M.D.,
and
Raymond Hull

HAWTHORN BOOKS, INC.
PUBLISHERS / NEW YORK

THE MALE CLIMACTERIC

Library of Congress Catalog Card Number: 74–18692

ISBN: 0–8015–4810–1

1 2 3 4 5 6 7 8 9 10

Contents

Introduction

SUMMER 1968

I begin to think I am going mad. I am walking down the Gower Point Road, chatting with an old friend, Don Cruikshank. He asks me a question. I know the answer, but I can't speak: My lips, jaws, and tongue won't move! After thirty seconds or so I regain control, but Don is looking at me oddly. This sort of thing has happened several times lately.

I am living alone in a country cottage, actually a former barn that I converted by my own labor into a little four-room house— two downstairs, two up in what used to be the hayloft. I am forty-nine years old, in first-class physical condition, and exceptionally strong and active for a man of my age. I cultivate a large vegetable garden. I carry driftwood from the beach on my back and saw it up for firewood, all with hand tools. I take a long walk every day.

I am a successful author, with all the work I want to do, a growing reputation, and a more-than-adequate income. This is, without doubt, the happiest, most rewarding period of my life.

Yet occasionally, for no reason I can discern, I have spells of desperate fear. I hardly dare climb the stairs to my bedroom at night. I make myself do it, then fling off my clothes and scramble into bed: I feel safer under the blankets. After a series of nightmares I wake up with a full bladder, still terrified; only with a great effort of will can I climb out of bed to urinate.

I usually have no difficulty with my work. On good days I write as much as 2,000 or 3,000 words of new material. Normally I sit down at the desk with a feeling of interest and eager anticipation.

But I have spells, lasting several days at a time, when I feel stupefied, unable to do any constructive thinking, unable to get on with my work.

During these spells my body temperature is severely upset: Feverish periods, when I'm drenched with sweat, alternate with periods of feeling bitterly cold, when I muffle myself in a sweater and heavy dressing gown to try and keep warm. One night in bed I sweated so much that I woke up and found the sheets soaked through; I had to get up and change them.

WHAT'S THE MATTER?

I am visiting Don Cruikshank in his cottage, sitting in the big old rocking chair near the door. I have another of those spells of near-unconsciousness; again I am unable to reply to a question of his.

"What's the matter with you lately, Ray?" he says. "You don't seem to be your usual self."

"It's nothing much," I answer. "It's a mild form of epilepsy called petit mal; it causes these little spells of faintness and then passes off again."

I had been reading medical books and discovered this "petit mal." It is indeed very much like what I've been feeling: The patient has a brief spell of faintness or giddiness, suddenly stops whatever he is doing, and in a few moments is back to normal. Some patients will pause in the middle of a sentence, stand silent a little while, and then continue, without knowing they had stopped. Many cases of petit mal do show periodicity: That is, the patient will be free of the symptoms for some time—a few days or a few weeks—and then will have some more of the spells. That fits me to a tee.

SEPTEMBER 1968

Another thing, and this seems to have no connection with petit mal: I've entirely lost my sex drive. In the past I had some good lovemaking sessions here in the barn; now I don't have the slightest desire for them. I couldn't get an erection for a thousand-dollar fee! Can it be my age? I don't *feel* old; I don't *look* old. Why this sudden onset of impotence?

September 8: J. V., a woman I knew when I lived in Vancouver, turns up in midafternoon, uninvited, unannounced, to visit me at the barn, carrying a brown paper bag containing her nightgown and toothbrush. I cook a nice dinner; we eat and talk pleasantly enough. But at night, she sleeps alone upstairs; I sleep downstairs. I don't know why she doesn't arouse me, and I'm ashamed to talk to her about it. She returns to town on the Sunday afternoon, leaving her nightgown behind. I wrap it up and mail it back to her. I suppose she feels insulted and won't return again.

WINTER 1968

I notice another strange symptom. I have a thick head of hair for my age, and my scalp has always been in healthy condition. Now, at intervals, I notice a heavy production of dandruff—very heavy, in fact. When I brush my hair, the flakes of dead skin shower to the floor like snow. This lasts for a few days at a time. Then begins a spell of the other symptoms—irrational fears, the hot and cold sweats, the so-called petit mal sensations, the brief feelings of going crazy—and within twenty-four hours the dandruff is gone and my scalp is as smooth as a baby's bottom.

I mentioned so-called petit mal. Since I talked to Don about it, I've read more on the subject and found that it is mainly a disease of childhood or young manhood, and almost never comes on after the age of thirty. So that probably leaves me out.

Why don't I go and see the doctor? It would take me several days to get an appointment, so by the time I see him, the symptoms will have passed off; I shall have nothing to show and will feel like a fool. Anyway, as soon as each spell is over, I feel fine, physically, emotionally, and mentally—I've never felt better—so I think there won't be another spell. Then, in a few weeks it starts all over again. Maybe I *am* going mad!

MARCH 1969

A couple of months ago I had what seemed to be an onset of rheumatism. There was stiffness and pain in the right knee and right elbow. It reached the point at which there was a constant, nagging pain; then came a big swelling of the knee and partial disability. I began to shrink from climbing the stairs because the knee hurt so much. I had to sit down to put on or take off my socks, pants, and shoes (I normally put them on standing up).

I became rather scared. This really seemed like old age coming on! I determined to improve my diet and began eating a lot of raw vegetable salads.

The results were amazing: Within two weeks all swelling and pain were gone. I am now beginning to feel an unaccustomed exhilaration for much of the day—a sensation of positive, bursting health that I have not known for years.

AUGUST 24, 1969

I went to Gibsons yesterday to see the bicycle race and the aquatic festival. I spent a good eight hours on my feet, never felt tired at all, and walking home (three miles) after 9 P.M. felt so full of pep that I had to *run* part of the way.

DECEMBER 1969

Recently rereading a book on diet, I realized that I had been neglecting vitamins. I got some vitamin A and some wheat-germ oil vitamin E and on November 30 began taking them regularly. I've also increased my intake of vitamin C.

JULY 1970

In May I returned to live in Vancouver. My general health continues to be good, but still, from time to time, I keep getting those bouts of strange symptoms, hot and cold spells, groundless fears, and so on. One good thing is that the spells of sweating and shivering are shorter than before—some last only a couple of minutes. I am also helped by the fact that I can go out, see a movie, converse at the Arts Club, or otherwise amuse myself, and so I don't brood over my own feelings as I had at Gibsons.

September 1970

The August 31 issue of *Time* contained a letter to the editor that briefly mentioned a "male climacteric," in which some middle-aged men experience symptoms much like those of the female menopause at more or less regular intervals, usually fifty-one to fifty-five days) Here is a clue. I will start to observe myself closely; I will record the dates when the unpleasant symptoms begin and when they stop. I want to see if there is any way to predict the onset of these spells.

The symptoms began on the afternoon of Saturday, September 5: alternate hot and cold spells, depression, brief feelings of going crazy, and gain of weight, apparently caused by water-retention, because I did not eat more than usual. The symptoms reached their height on Monday, September 7, and had almost disappeared by the afternoon of Wednesday, September 9. During this time I felt unable to think clearly or act decisively. I could do no useful writing, although I did some reading. I did not feel much like meeting or talking to people.

The Cycle

A year's self-observation showed that, for me, there was indeed a cycle: a few days' symptoms, then several weeks' excellent health and normal good spirits, then another spell of symptoms.

The length of the cycle varied somewhat, but averaged forty-five days.

I bought a clinical thermometer and began taking my temperature each morning immediately after getting dressed. I found that on the day symptoms began the temperature was up, high above normal. Immediately after the symptoms disappeared, the temperature dropped, then oscillated about normal until the onset of the next spell.

There was a noticeable emotional cycle, too. Normally I am of a placid, equable disposition (I was, as a young man, profoundly influenced by the Stoic philosophers); several times friends have criticized me for showing too little emotion about people and events. Yet during the spells of symptoms, my temperament is entirely changed: I feel depressed—about myself, my work, my friends, the whole human race. I am watching myself in these prolonged moods of depression; I'm aware that they don't express my normal self; I'm making notes on how I feel, on what I think and what I do; and I'm wondering how such mood changes affect other men.

This depression is unpleasant; but there is another emotional effect that is dangerous. On any trivial provocation I may switch from the depressed, apathetic mood, to one of near-insane rage. For example, about 10 P.M. on February 26, 1971, I was walking home from the Arts Club. There had been a light snowfall earlier in the evening, and I was carrying a folded umbrella. Outside the Blue Horizon Hotel four young men were throwing snowballs at one another. A snowball came within a few feet of me. Normally I would have laughed and walked on. Now I flew into a fury, lifted my umbrella like a club, and rushed at the man who had thrown the snowball. He grabbed the umbrella and threatened to break it. His three friends stood by, watching. After a minute of hard looks and heavy breathing, the two of us separated; he rejoined the snowball game, and I walked on home, trembling. Once again, I had been watching myself, thinking: My God! Suppose I'd been carrying some weapon more lethal than an umbrella! Suppose those other three men had set upon me and beaten me up!

One more thing: Just at the time when, after a few days, the symptoms pass off, I'm in an extraordinarily mirthful mood; I will howl with laughter over someone's little witticism, over a book, or the radio—something that normally would barely raise a smile. This elated mood lasts for perhaps a few hours; then I settle back into my normal calm, easygoing temperament for another five or six weeks, until the next spell of physical symptoms and depression begins.

Unpleasant Effects

There were sudden spells of what I must call "paralysis of the will." On January 22, 1971, I was checking out of the Lord Simcoe Hotel in Toronto. I was at the cashier's desk with pen in hand, ready to sign some travelers' checks to pay my bill and on came one of these spells. *I could not sign my name.* I struggled with the pen for a few seconds; the right hand would not move. I had to mutter an apology, step aside, let a couple more guests check out, and wait till I recovered control of my hand. For me, in these circumstances, this was simply embarrassing. But for other men, in different circumstances—a surgeon in a critical operation or a general at the decisive moment of a battle—it could be disastrous!

I do not have what one would call an outstandingly good memory, yet most of the time I get through my work and my social life without any serious difficulties. During the spells of symptoms, however, I have sudden, inexplicable lapses of memory.

In the spring of 1971 I was writing a collaborative biography of Gassy Jack Deighton, one of the pioneer settlers of Vancouver. For some months I had been working on it with Olga Ruskin, a writer living in West Vancouver, constantly meeting her for discussions, writing notes back and forth, telephoning, and interchanging installments of the script. On the morning of Monday, May 24, I wrote her a letter enclosing some notes on the script, sealed it, stamped it, and laid it on the bookcase to take with me when I went out for the morning paper. At 11:30 I was ready to go out. I saw the letter, picked it up, read the name and address on it, but could not, to save my life, have said what was in it, or who was this Olga Ruskin to whom it was addressed. I was about to open it to see what it contained when, by checking through the files on my desk, I found the carbon copies of the letter and enclosures. I could not honestly say that, even then, I "remembered"—rather I "realized" what must be in the envelope.

On August 26, 1971, I was dining at Maureen's apartment, with her and Jo-Anne. Suddenly, I had one of these spells of amnesia. As I sat there eating, drinking, and talking, *I forgot their names!* I observed myself trying to remember and failing. If I'd had my diary handy, I could have consulted it to remind myself; but it was in my jacket, and Maureen had taken that away and hung it up before dinner. So all evening I had to do my best to maintain a conversation, without knowing whom I was talking to!

Here again, in these circumstances, the experience was merely annoying to me. The other two were talkative enough; the evening was not spoiled. But suppose I had been a lawyer defending a murderer in court. Suppose I had been a politician, making a major policy statement in the legislature. I don't have to suppose: I now know that many other middle-aged men undergo similar mental lapses, and they cannot all get off so lightly as I do.

Another time I was at a television station to do an interview to promote a new book of mine. I had arrived early, so was waiting over a cup of coffee in the cafeteria for show time. I had another of these memory lapses and forgot the name of the show, the name of the interviewer, the title of the book—everything that I was there for. By great good fortune, my memory returned a few minutes before show time, and the interview went off smoothly. But suppose my memory had *not* returned!

Here's a disturbing physical experience: October 7, 1971, at 10:55 A.M., I was walking through the underground shopping arcade of the Toronto-Dominion Bank building in Toronto. I had a sudden spell of faintness and dizziness. I managed to keep walking, but retained my balance only by conscious effort, as if I were drunk. After about a minute, the dizziness passed off as suddenly

as it began. Here again, for me, there were no serious conse-
quences. But suppose I had been climbing a mountain, driving a
bus, or flying an airplane.

IMPROVEMENT

I continued for two years, keeping records and trying to build
up my health by exercise, a nutritious diet, and plenty of supple-
mentary vitamins. Here are some excerpts from my notes.

January 10, 1973: "Another period began on January 4, but
with notable differences from previous ones. The interval since the
last period was longer than ever before—fifty-seven days. The
previous longest interval was fifty-three days, the average to date,
forty-four.

"The symptoms were so much milder than formerly that at
first I could not be sure whether it was one of the usual periods.
There were no hot flashes or sweating, no insomnia, no bad
dreams, and no spells of bad temper.

"The only physical symptom was one short dizzy spell on the
5th. But I experienced a slight sluggishness in thinking, and the
usual lapses of memory. One amusing instance was when I went
to the Fine Arts Cinema to see *Travels with My Aunt*. Only after
the film had been running several minutes did I remember that I
had seen it a few days earlier!

"I'm just about back to normal now."

July 22, 1973: "Many hairs of my head are turning from white
to dark. Those very old scars on my legs are healing up. My
memory is noticeably improving."

October 1973: "I spoke at Kitchener, Ontario, at a conference,
Perspectives on Paperbacks. It went over very well. There was a
wine and cheese party after the lecture. I woke up next morning in
bed with a pretty young woman. Unfortunately, as it turned out,
I had been too drunk to make love to her. (A moral here: libido
fully restored by now, but potency temporarily destroyed by
alcohol!)"

RESEARCH

I began interviewing middle-aged men. Some of them were having much the same experience as I was; what impressed me was their profound relief at being able to talk about it. Each of them had thought that he was suffering alone; to discover that the experience was not uncommon, to be assured that he was not going mad, to hear down-to-earth, prosaic Raymond Hull talk about his symptoms, his experiences, his former fears—that was a great comfort to them.

I had questionnaires printed and began passing them out to men and women who, in conversation, admitted to some degree of experience with the subject. Many of the replies yielded fascinating material. The following is a replica of the form I used.

I am investigating the so-called male climacteric, or change of life, during which many men (usually somewhere in their forties or fifties) undergo a noticeable transformation in health, temperament, and sexual behavior. I should be grateful for your observations on this subject. Names will not be used. (Signed) Raymond Hull.

1. Can you think of any instances from history, legend, or literature where men showed a sudden transformation at this time of life? Please give details.
2. Do you personally know of any similar example? No _____ Yes _____
    (a) Who was it? Yourself? _____ Your husband? _____ Someone else? (Please indicate the relationship) _____
    - (b) At what age did the change begin?
    - (c) What were the physical symptoms?
    - (d) What were the most obvious changes of behavior toward family, friends, work, etc.?
3. In some men the physical symptoms and behavior changes recur at more or less regular intervals. Was that so in this case?
    - (a) If so, what, roughly, was the interval from one spell to the next?
    - (b) Did there seem to be any outside influence that would

"trigger" a spell of the physical symptoms or of the changed behavior? If so, what was it?

4. Did the man take any medical or other treatment?
   (a) If so, what? For how long? What results did it produce?
   (b) If not, why not?
5. Was the "change of life" permanent? Yes _____ No _____ If not, at what age did the man's health and behavior return to normal?

THE SEARCH FOR A COLLABORATOR

I realized that to write a successful, authoritative book on this subject, I should find a collaborator with medical qualifications.

I spoke first to a doctor friend of mine. He seemed keenly interested; he was going through the change of life himself, with symptoms even more severe than mine. I asked him about testosterone therapy (test-ost'-er-ōn: the most important of the male hormones or androgens). He said it was certainly effective but so terribly dangerous that he would never use it on himself or prescribe it for a patient. I saw him at a party on a Sunday evening in December 1971 and arranged to meet him again the following Wednesday for our first conference on the project. We never conferred: He went home from that party, put a rifle in his mouth, and blew his head off.

In mid-1972 I found another doctor who was interested in the subject. He searched the library of the local medical association and lent me all the books that mentioned the male climacteric. (A scanty collection: I read the material in one afternoon.) My own symptoms were already growing milder. Before they disappeared altogether, I wanted to try the effect of testosterone injections. The doctor said that the next time I felt the onset of the symptoms I should hurry to his office; he would give me the testosterone injection and we would see the effect it produced— interesting material for the book and, according to him, no risk at all. But he never administered the injection: Before my next spell of symptoms occurred, he had died of a heart attack.

His successor seemed interested in my project but was against the use of testosterone, "especially as you are getting over it by yourself." He dropped some hints about psychosomatic causes— the realization that one is over the hill and has not much to look forward to, etc., etc. I did not explain to him that, in my case, these symptoms had coincided with what was by far the most successful and satisfying period of my life. Anyway, before I could make any progress with this physician, he abandoned the practice and moved away. I never saw or heard of him again.

Still searching for a collaborator, I got an introduction to a man in the Department of Medicine at the University of British Columbia. I had to wait three weeks for an interview. It was brief: He received me coolly and said that he certainly would not be interested in my project, because there is no such phenomenon as a male change of life.

Continuing the search, I renewed an old acquaintance with Helmut Ruebsaat. Years before, we had both been performing members of a folk-song club. He already was familiar with the subject and shared my feelings of its importance. Shortly thereafter we began the collaboration that produced this book.

Many people who completed questionnaires, wrote letters, and gave interviews to provide material for this book did so with the understanding that their names would not be revealed. Statements preceded by "A man said," "A woman reports," and examples in which identities are concealed by initials are drawn from this confidential material.

From here on, Dr. Ruebsaat speaks in the first person.

Raymond Hull
Vancouver, B.C.

Part I

EFFECTS OF

THE CLIMACTERIC

The male climacteric is a critical stage, a turning point in the lives of men. Many men—usually somewhere between the years of forty-five and sixty—undergo major physical and emotional changes that produce severe disruptions of their health, their careers, and their private lives.

Chapter 1 describes in detail the sexual, general physical, and emotional symptoms of the climacteric. These symptoms are unpleasant enough for the man who experiences them, yet they have further effects: They change his feelings and his conduct toward other people, and they change other people's feelings and conduct toward him. In Chapters 2 and 3 I shall describe how the climacteric affects the man's home life, his work, and his general behavior in society. A glossary at the back of the book explains the meanings of technical terms.

1
The Symptoms

Many men pass fairly smoothly from adolescence to maturity, to middle age, and to old age. By clock and calendar they keep track of the hours and days; yet they experience no abrupt bodily transitions, no physical mileposts on the road: There is no occasion on which the man is forced to say, "I am noticeably not the same man I was three months ago."

For a woman the situation is different: Each menstrual period gives her an uncompromising reminder that time is passing. The woman also must expect to reach a major milepost. More or less suddenly she will stop menstruating; her ovaries will no longer release eggs and will diminish their production of the feminizing hormone estrogen. She may experience a few, or many, of a galaxy of physical and emotional symptoms associated with the menopause. After the menopause, she is certainly not the same woman she was before. Her life, in some respects, may be more enjoyable now, but her reproductive ability is gone forever.

Some men do *not* pass smoothly through the stages from maturity to middle age and old age. In some cases the man's physical, mental, and emotional equilibrium is suddenly deranged. He cannot help noticing the change; it frightens him. In other cases there is no such sudden change: The man himself does not perceive that anything is happening to him, although his family, friends, and fellow workers notice he has changed.

This change, whether sudden or gradual, is manifested by various symptoms, many of which resemble the symptoms of the menopause, and it is usually associated with a major disruption of the man's sex life. For these reasons it has sometimes been called "the male menopause."

There are three reasons why I do not intend to use the term menopause in this book with reference to men. First, the word "menopause" (derived from the Greek *menos*, which means a month) signifies the cessation of some function formerly occurring at monthly intervals. But in the male there is no recognizable monthly sexual or hormonal cycle—nothing comparable to the female menses. The normal man does not have fertile and infertile periods: He produces millions of sperm every day. So it is wrong to imply, by using the phrase "male menopause," the former existence of a monthly cycle that has now ceased.

Second, the change in men also differs from the menopause in women because, as I said earlier, many men never experience it. Even for the men who do, this midlife change does not necessarily end their reproductive lives, for in men the change can be reversible—another difference from woman's menopause. In some cases the symptoms pass off after awhile without any treatment; the men regain their former physical, mental and sexual abilities. In other cases the change would be permanent but, by appropriate medical or psychiatric treatment, most of them can obtain considerable relief or complete cure: The disagreeable symptoms are reduced or eliminated; the men regain their interest in and enjoyment of sex; and their reproductive capability may be prolonged far into old age.

Third, a major problem in dealing with these changes—a problem for wives, employers, and physicians—is to get men to admit that something is wrong with them and then to accept advice and treatment. To write and talk about a "male menopause" is for many men an insult to their masculinity, an implication that they are womanish, sissified. Why, then, make what is already a difficult situation even more difficult by one's choice of words?

A word that aptly describes the condition is "climacteric" (an anglicized form of the medical term *climacterium*, which is derived from the Greek *klimakter*, which means the rung of a ladder), meaning a major change, a turning point in human life.* (There are two acceptable pronunciations of climacteric: klī-mak'-ter-ik or klī-mak-ter'-ik.)

Now let us see how this climacteric, this midlife crisis, may change the lives of the men who go through it. There are a number of characteristic symptoms, although of course not every man will experience all of them. Before I describe the symptoms in detail, I want to make two points that are essential to a clear understanding of what follows.

THE PSYCHOSOMATIC RELATIONSHIP

The word "psychosomatic" is derived from the Greek words *psyche* (life, mind, or soul) and *soma* (body). It refers to the intricate interdependence, the functional unity, between man's central nervous system (the "seat" of his mind) and the rest of the human organism. The term is a fairly new one; its current acceptance indicates the reversal of a centuries-old misconception.

According to the traditional dualistic concept, man was divided into two separate entities—the soul or mind and the body. One temporarily lived inside the other, like a man in a house, yet there was no close bond between them: The house might be demolished, but the man could go on and live elsewhere.

Dualism had been dominant in Eastern thought since the time of Zoroaster (630–541 B.C.), who influenced Plato (c. 427–347 B.C.) and his disciple Aristotle (384–322 B.C.). It taught that the body was of less worth than the spirit and therefore should be subject to it. This dualistic theory has crept into the Judeo-Christian philosophy, and still exerts a widespread influence today. I do not intend to argue for or against the survival of the human spirit or personality after death, but I will say emphatically that the mind and body are *not* separate entities during life.

---

* "Climacteric" is an adjective as well as a noun, so we can correctly say that the man who is experiencing the male climacteric is a climacteric male.

It is generally understood that physical pain or illness may have a depressing effect on the mind; yet many people do not realize how often psychological events produce the symptoms and signs of what might seem to be purely physical disorders. Psychosomatic diseases are bodily dysfunctions caused by a special, abnormal way of responding to difficulties in living.

Research on the autonomic nervous system and the brain has established definite pathways related to emotions. Under normal, healthy conditions psychic energy created by emotions travels along these pathways to express the person's feelings in terms of action. (For example, if a person is frightened, a natural reaction is to run away.)

The switchboard, or bridge, for mind-body connections appears to be the hypothalamus (hī-po-thal′-a-mus), located in the mid-brain or diencephalon (dī-en-sef′-a-lon), which organizes the motor (muscular), visceral (inner organ), and glandular responses to emotional experiences. Emotional conflicts, or severe emotional stress, may generate excessive currents of psychic energy that can upset the switchboard and become "short-circuited" into the autonomic nervous system.

The autonomic nervous system regulates bodily functions that are outside conscious control—for example, the actions of the heart and the digestive organs. It consists of two subsystems—the sympathetic and parasympathetic. Both the sympathetic and parasympathetic subsystems can be utilized as "lightning rods" for the electrically overloaded central nervous system.

For an example of how the process works, consider a man who is subject to many small emotional irritations, say from a constantly nagging coworker. His suppressed reactions could build up an energy potential, like a tightly wound alarm clock, that may be triggered at an inopportune moment by some apparently trivial stimulus.

The man may take some action to relieve the psychic pressure: He may have a fight over the issue; he may run away; or he may start negotiations to solve the problem. Any of these courses would, as it were, open the safety valve. But if he does not do *something*, the psychic energy may be short-circuited along the vagus nerve into his digestive system, and there create spasms of stomach cramps, or if the psychic short circuit goes to the respiratory system, the man may develop bronchial asthma.

There is good evidence that middle age is a particularly vulnerable time of life for development of such symptoms in men: Stomach cramps and asthma are only two of many. Other psychosomatic symptoms commonly seen in middle-aged males are peptic ulcers, hot flashes, excessive sweating, heart palpitations, angina (an-jīn′-a) or pseudoangina, certain forms of high blood pressure, skin conditions, impotence, premature ejaculation, and headaches (including migraines).

As another illustration of the intricate mind-body interrelation, let me offer the case history of a family that used to be in my care. Mr. and Mrs. C. S. had a daughter aged sixteen and two sons aged thirteen and six. They were members of an extreme fundamentalist religious sect; one of the sect's teachings was that a "born-again Christian" was no longer capable of feeling such emotions as hostility or resentment, particularly toward his own kin. Yet this family became entrapped (unknown to themselves) in a severe love-hate conflict that produced extremely destructive effects on their health.

The mother was a compulsive, obsessive, dominating personality; she absolutely smothered everybody in the family with her brand of love. She talked incessantly, made all decisions, and did everything for everybody. She believed that she was demonstrating complete dedication to the service of her family. In reality her husband and the children were made to feel helpless, dependent, inadequate, and inferior. They tried to love her, yet, to use a significant colloquialism, they hated her guts but would not allow themselves to admit it.

These were the results of this emotional suppression:

1. The father developed bronchial asthma attacks and ended up in the hospital (one way to get away from it all).

2. The sixteen-year-old daughter suffered hysterical deafness (not just the "mother-deafness" that pediatricians know so well).

3. The thirteen-year-old son developed a stomach ulcer.

4. The six-year-old son, who had been toilet-trained, began to dirty his pants again.

5. The mother herself relapsed into her peptic ulcer disease.

This is an unusually large gamut of psychosomatic disease to find in one family at the same time.

I emphasize, then, that in psychosomatic illnesses the symptoms express the response of the *whole person*, the mind-body entity, to changing events, both external and internal—for example, to someone else's nagging (external) or to one's own worrying (internal).

I felt it was necessary to make this brief mention of the psychosomatic relationship here, near the start of the book. In Chapter 5 I shall give a more detailed description of the typical psychosomatic factors of the male climacteric. In the rest of this chapter I shall describe the characteristic symptoms of the male climacteric.

SEXUAL SYMPTOMS

The accepted "normal" pattern for a man's sexual ability and interest can be depicted graphically by a curve that rises to a peak at about age eighteen and then begins a very slow decline. This is what many men actually experience; they continue with a moderate, yet satisfying, sexual activity far into old age. Some men are less fortunate: Somewhere in middle age they experience a more or less severe disruption of their sex lives.

Decline or Loss of Potency

Potency is the ability to achieve an erection and sustain it long enough to perform the sexual act to the satisfaction of both partners. Erection is accomplished by blood congestion of three sponge-like cavernous spaces that surround the long urinary passage in the shaft and head of the penis. Tiny muscles constrict the veins that normally carry blood out of the penis, thus trapping the blood that the arteries are pumping into it. The spongy tissues swell, the penis increases in thickness and length, and stands up stiffly. Soon after ejaculation, the muscles relax, the veins expand, blood congestion in the penis is reduced, and it becomes limp again (called detuminescence or resolution).

These muscular contractions and relaxations are not under conscious control (although many men have wished that they were). They are directed by reflexes in the autonomic nervous system. A man may curse this erection mechanism when it gives him an erection at an inconvenient time; otherwise he seldom thinks of it, except when he is overanxious about his sexual performance at a specific moment. This acute anxiety, known as fear of erectile failure, not uncommonly occurs on wedding nights, leaving the groom dismayed and the bride puzzled, but the problem usually resolves itself once this formidable occasion has passed. It must be distinguished from true impotence.

Primary Impotence

Primary impotence is a condition in which a man has never in his life been able to achieve an erection because of some anatomical or hormonal abnormality. Primary impotence is not the condition we are concerned with here; where it exists, it should have been diagnosed and if possible treated long before middle age.

Secondary Impotence

Secondary impotence, much more common than primary impotence, is the condition in which a man who has previously been able to produce an erection suffers a partial or total loss of that ability. This secondary, or acquired, impotence can show itself in four forms.

1. Permanent loss of potency.

The affected man never gets an erection at any time. I shall discuss this condition at some length later in the book, but there is one point I would like to make immediately, before readers form any false notions. This type of impotence may indeed be permanent if the man simply resigns himself to it and makes no attempt to get treatment. But he should *not* resign himself. Theoretically, any man who has previously had satisfactory sexual experiences can, under proper treatment, regain the ability to get, and use, an erection; this applies even if the man has been castrated! He may require physiological, psychological, or hormonal treatment, but with such treatment there are excellent prospects for full recovery.

2. *Temporary or periodical impotence.*

In this condition the man can produce an erection and achieve intercourse some of the time, but at other times he cannot. I said earlier that a man may expect a gradual decline of potency, a gradual reduction in frequency of intercourse as he ages; but any sudden, considerable decline in erectile potency or frequency should be taken as a significant symptom. Of course, there may be an obvious physical or emotional reason for it—for example, some illness, severe business worries, or a quarrel with the spouse. But in such cases the condition should clear itself up when the cause disappears.

3. *Weak or short-lasting erection.*

This problem, like fear of erectile failure, is not uncommon in early life, particularly on a man's first sexual encounter with a new woman. But sometimes a man in middle life, after years of satisfactory sexual experiences, finds that this loss of erection is occurring often or even every time he attempts intercourse. He gets an erection, but it is not hard enough to penetrate the vagina, or he may lose his erection just in the act of penetration. The psychological factors involved in this form of impotence are discussed in Chapter 5.

4. *Premature ejaculation.*

The man gets an erection, but before he penetrates, or in some cases just as he penetrates, he ejaculates. The penis promptly falls limp, and the man must withdraw.

All four of these potency disturbances are aggravated by fear of erectile failure. For example, suppose the man notices that he has for a considerable time had no erection at all; or that he has been having intermittent spells of impotence; or that he now sometimes loses his erection before penetration; or that he now usually has a premature ejaculation. Tonight he is going to make another attempt at intercourse. Naturally he is anxious; he thinks, "This time will I be able to do it properly?" And, naturally, *the fear* of another failure *increases the probability* of another failure.

Impotence and Sterility

Perhaps I should emphasize that loss of potency is not the same thing as sterility. Sterility is the failure to produce living sperm. A man may be fully potent and yet be sterile. He can enjoy satisfying intercourse as often as he wants it, yet he cannot father a child because he produces too few or no sperm or because the sperm he produces are dead or otherwise defective. On the other hand, a man may have suffered complete loss of potency and yet still be producing a normal number of live sperm. He is impotent, but fertile. In most cases, there is no physical relationship between these two conditions.

Loss of Libido

Libido (lib-eed'-o or lib'-id-o), from the Latin word meaning desire, is the desire for sexual activity. Some psychologists (among them the Freudians) would give a much wider meaning to the word, suggesting that libido is the principal driving force of life and that in the male all creative human activity is unconsciously related to the urge to mate. This view of libido, I feel, belittles man; on this theory (to paraphrase Samuel Butler's aphorism on hens), a man is only a sperm's way of making another sperm. However, this chapter is not the place to argue the purpose of human existence; I just want to define my terms. I am using "libido" in the narrow sense as defined above.

There is not necessarily any connection between libido and potency. Many men, though impotent, desire sexual intercourse; and some men, though not impotent, lose, intermittently or completely, all desire for sex. (For factors influencing libido, see Chapter 5.)

A man described this experience.

> I'm forty-eight now, and I recall it starting about four years ago. I should explain that sexual activity has always been a great factor in my life. Through my life I've made love to a number of women. Eleven years ago I got married, and from then on I didn't look at or touch another woman.
>
> The change began very slowly, and I was puzzled by it. The most salient feature of this was that I would lose sexual drive. I used to have no interest in touching—especially touching—my wife, and of starting anything that might lead to intercourse, to the point where our relationship became quite stressed.
>
> We went to a psychiatrist (originally for another reason), and he suggested all kinds of physical stimulation, to which I replied that I wasn't interested, and I couldn't change this around: There was no way in which I would be interested in physically touching my wife.

The couple separated and were divorced; the man went to live with another woman but said, "even with her, where there were no sexual hangups such as I thought I had with my wife, I found periods during which, although I appeared to love her very much, I couldn't stand being close to her: it was sometimes too much for me, sharing the same bed with her."

Changed Sex Life

For many middle-aged men the sex life has become just as much a matter of habit as the journey to work, the daily newspaper, or the nightly walk with the dog. The Friday night intercourse is no more—perhaps less—exciting than the Saturday night poker game. Yet at the climacteric this habit, too, may be broken.

Some men, after years of marital fidelity, suddenly begin chasing other women, particularly women much younger than themselves.

One man said that he had "a yearning for a final romantic love affair 'ere the end, with someone younger but not inexperienced." Another man said, "Before I go, I want to have the experience of a true love relationship. Without that, my life would be incomplete." A woman described her husband as "finding relationships with other women and having no further sexual interest at home." Still another man reported his own "frequent disastrous involvements with younger women, where the authority of age and position is used as power play. Panic when affairs become too serious."

Some men undergo radical changes in their sex lives. There have recently been reported several cases in which men at an age when they may well have been experiencing the climacteric have renounced masculinity altogether and have undergone sex-change surgery. Other men, to all appearances heterosexual, will at the climacteric turn to homosexuality.

OTHER PHYSICAL SYMPTOMS

Now I will describe some physical symptoms of the climacteric that do not directly involve the man's sex life. We cannot, of course, divide a man into sections, separated from each other like a ship's water-tight compartments: The whole man is affected, all the time, by the efficient or faulty operation of each of his bodily and mental functions. For example, if he suffers frequent, severe headaches, his work, his social life, and his sex life will be impaired. Conversely, a full, satisfying sex life tends to enrich every other aspect of his life.

I will describe the physical symptoms of the climacteric one at a time, but please bear in mind that in many cases several different symptoms may be manifestations of the same underlying problem.

Urinary Irregularities

The kidneys filter the blood, removing waste products and surplus water and minerals from the body in the form of urine. Urine passes from the kidneys through two tubes, the ureters, to the bladder, a muscle-walled sac that gradually expands to store the urine until the filled bladder urges one to urinate. At this time, the sphincter (sfink'-ter), a ring of muscle at the outlet of the bladder, relaxes. The bladder muscles contract, and urine flows down the urethra (you-reeth'-ra), a tube that passes through the prostate gland and the penis. Normally, the stream of urine is forceful, the pressure being applied by muscular contraction of the bladder. The flow continues uninterrupted until the bladder is empty and then stops cleanly.

Childhood bladder training consists of developing voluntary control over this sphincter; some children achieve this control more easily than others. Even in a healthy adult, sphincter control can be lost, under such influences as alcoholic intoxication or a paroxysm of mirth.

The average output of urine for adults is three to five pints a day; the output for an individual may vary considerably according to the amount of liquid he drinks and to the amount of water he loses through the skin by perspiration (the unnoticed evaporation of water) or sweating (perceptible excretion of salt solution).

The bladder can comfortably store a pint or more of urine, so normally one urinates only four to six times a day. Urine production does not proceed at a uniform rate; most of it is produced, and voided, during the morning and early afternoon. The man in good health does not have to urinate during the night, unless he has drunk an unusually large volume of liquids during the evening.

The urinary flow may be disturbed at the climacteric due to enlargement of the prostate gland, which surrounds the urinary passage at the bladder outlet. (This enlargement is probably due to hormonal changes.) The man urinates more often than he used to—up to eight or ten times a day. He may have to get up once, or several times, during the night to urinate. The stream of urine becomes weaker and maybe thin or diverted. There may be dribbling or hesitancy before the flow begins and then several stoppages and resumptions of the flow before the bladder is empty. There may also be some dribbling of urine after the man thought he had finished.

The onset of this condition is very gradual; the man scarcely notices anything until the symptoms are well advanced. (Despite these problems, the climacteric male does succeed in emptying his bladder. Retention of urine in the bladder usually occurs with advanced cases of prostate enlargement in older men.)

Fluid Retention (Swelling)

A healthy man's body is, by weight, more than half water. His heart, arteries, capillaries, and veins contain about ten pints of blood, which is mostly water. All the cells of which his body is made contain intracellular fluid—water solutions of various minerals—which make up 24 to 38 percent of the body's weight. Filling the minute spaces between the cells is the extracellular fluid, about 24 percent of body weight.

The cells absorb minerals and nutrients from the extracellular fluid and excrete waste into it by diffusion through the cell walls. The kidneys are mainly responsible for the eventual removal of these dissolved waste products. The kidneys also play a large part in controlling the total amount of water in the body: More liquid consumed means more urine passed, as every beer-drinker knows.

When one is in good health, this balance of liquids in the body is accurately maintained. But the deterioration of blood circulation caused by age can upset the complicated fluid-control system, as can the hormone changes of the climacteric. We do not know all the details of the mechanism by which these hormone changes affect the fluid-control system; but there is some disturbance of the dissolved mineral content of the tissue fluid. There is a reduced output of urine, particularly during the latter part of the day, and

—this is the obvious symptom—tissue fluid tends to accumulate in certain parts of the body.

During the day, when the man is standing or sitting, the influence of gravity can cause fluid accumulations in the feet and ankles, the hands, and the lower rump. The man's shoes begin to hurt him; the band of his wristwatch or his ring begins to cut into the swollen skin; or his pants begin to feel unusually tight.

During the night, while the man is lying down, the pressure of fluid in these parts is reduced. The kidneys can now do their work more efficiently, and by morning the swellings have disappeared; but by midafternoon, they are back again. (This fluid retention, by the way, is less common in middle-aged men than in women.)

Hot Flashes

During hot flashes, the man feels uncomfortably hot; often his face is flushed. As a rule, this hot feeling comes on quickly, in the space of a few seconds. The hot flash may last anywhere from a few seconds to several hours and may be accompanied by sweating. It may subside gradually or may pass off as quickly as it began. The man may then return to a normal temperature sensation, feeling neither hot nor cold, or he may pass straight from the hot flash into a cold spell, a shorter or longer time of feeling unpleasantly chilly.

Here is how one man described this symptom: "I would have strong perspiration and yet a feeling of cold, especially in the extremities. These attacks usually lasted three to five hours; I usually felt very uncomfortable during this time." Another man said, "I would notice an increased flow of perspiration under the arms, running down at the side of the rib cage." Another: "With me, the cold feeling usually comes first, then the hot. The sweating is particularly noticeable at night; sometimes my bed sheets have been soaked through with sweat."

Let us see what is happening here. Body temperature normally stays within a range of about 1° Fahrenheit, fluctuating daily from a low point in the early hours of the morning to a high point in early evening. The temperature-regulation system is controlled by the hypothalamus, a small area in the floor of the midbrain.

If body temperature tends to rise—for example, by excessive heat in the environment, by wearing too many clothes, by hard physical exercise, or by fever—an extra blood supply appears in the capillaries, the tiny blood vessels of the skin. The capillaries are dilated; consequently the skin becomes flushed and radiates more heat to the surrounding air. If this method is not sufficient to reduce the body temperature, the sweat glands of the skin abundantly excrete their dilute salt solution (the evaporation of this liquid uses up a lot of body heat). Conversely, if the body becomes cold, the skin capillaries shrink, and the skin turns pale and radiates less heat; sweat production is reduced.

Messages from the hypothalamus to the capillaries and sweat glands are conveyed by the vasomotor (vaz'-o-motor) nerves, a part of the autonomic nervous system responsible for enlarging and reducing the diameter of blood vessels and thus varying the supply of blood to different parts of the body according to need. Sometimes, though, the vasomotor nerves start working when there is no real need to increase or decrease the blood flow; such irregularities are called "vasomotor disturbances." For example, rage or shame may produce flushing of the skin; grief may turn it pale; fear may produce a pale skin and a cold sweat. Hormonal changes, too, can produce vasomotor disturbances—flushing, sweating, and chilly feelings quite unrelated to the temperature of the environment or to the amount of clothing one is wearing.

This is what is happening during the hot flashes and chilly spells of the climacteric. There is rarely, if ever, an objective rise or fall of body temperature that is measurable by the thermometer. But the autonomic nerve fibers controlling the blood vessels are "out of tune," so the capillary circulation at the body surface is suddenly increased or decreased and the man feels hot or cold.

Heart Symptoms

Most people do not notice the incessant beating of their hearts, except, perhaps, after a spell of brisk exercise. But the man at the climacteric may become aware of his own heartbeats: He often feels the pounding sensation in his chest; in quiet surroundings— in bed at night, for example—he actually hears it.

He may also have spells of paroxysmal tachycardia (par-ok-siz'-mal tak-i-kard'-i-a) when, without any of the usual causes— hard exercise, fever, alcohol, fear, and so on—the heartbeat accelerates much above its usual rate of 60 to 70 beats per minute. It may go as high as 160 to 200 beats per minute. He may also experience irregular heartbeat—rapid variations in the pulse and heartbeat or missed beats. All these symptoms are usually caused by chronic mental or emotional stress.

Pseudoangina

The man may feel a sharp pain in the front center of his chest, or on the left side, much like that of angina pectoris. Real angina pectoris is caused by an inadequate supply of oxygen to the heart muscle, which then goes into a painful state of metabolic starvation. Angina is brought on by physical or mental exertion. The pain often radiates along the arteries to the left shoulder and arm and sometimes to the neck and back. It is usually relieved by rest or by nitroglycerin tablets.

The pseudoangina pain is not caused by any defect of the heart; it is almost never brought on by physical exertion. Its most common cause is chronic anxiety. It cannot be relieved by rest or nitroglycerin, but usually responds to sedation. Another common cause of pseudoangina in middle-aged men is neuralgia or myalgia (muscle pain) due to strain of the intervertebral joints—the joints between the segments of the backbone—or to disease of the intervertebral disks—the gristly pads that separate the segments of the backbone.

Peptic Ulcers

Middle-aged men are a high-risk group for development of ulcers of the esophagus (gullet), stomach, and duodenum (the first 9 inches of the small intestine that adjoin the stomach). Excessive production of hydrochloric acid in the stomach, beyond what is normally needed for digestion, and spastic contractions of esophagus, stomach, and duodenum lead to damage of the mucous membranes that line these parts of the digestive tract. First there is a chronic inflammation, followed by the formation of the open sores called ulcers. The ulcer patient suffers intermittent pain somewhere in the upper abdomen, usually temporarily relieved after eating. He may also feel nauseated from time to time.

Itching and Formication

Most of the time, we are not conscious of the various sensations that are experienced by the skin and transmitted to the brain—the pressure of the buttocks on a chair, for example, or the pressure of the fingers on a book. Itching is a localized sensation strong enough to force itself upon the attention; the natural reaction to an itch is to scratch it.

Itching may be felt in two different forms: Local pruritus (proor-ī'-tus) continues in the same area or areas; formication (from *formica,* the Latin word for ant) feels like insects crawling on or under the skin, causing a sensation of tickling or stinging rather than an itch.

These sensations may vary in intensity from person to person and from time to time. The irritation may be so mild that the man can forget it simply by diverting his mind to something else. In severe cases, the man scratches until he draws blood, can scarcely think of anything but the itching by day, and can get no sleep at night.

Pruritus and formication, like hot flashes, are caused by disturbances of the autonomic nervous system. They are usually entirely subjective. Rarely is there any rash or inflammation, except for the skin damage caused by scratching. In some cases, however, there may be a rash caused by allergies, hives, or atopic skin reactions. (An atopic reaction is an oversensitive response to skin irritation, locally or elsewhere than at the point where the rash appears—for example, in response to something eaten or inhaled.)

There is no characteristic duration or frequency for itching or formication: One man may itch occasionally and briefly; another for a few hours only on certain days; a third may itch all day and every day. There is no characteristic location: One man may have pruritus all over his body; another may get formication only in certain areas. Each patient has his own subjective experience and description.

These symptoms may seem vaguely amusing to people who have never felt them; yet they can cause suffering that is intense and prolonged enough to drive a man almost to the point of suicide.

Air Hunger

Normally the breathing process is carried on unconsciously: The frequency and depth of the breaths are automatically regulated by the respiratory center in the brain to maintain the correct proportions of oxygen and carbon dioxide in the blood. A healthy man, sitting down, breathes about fifteen to eighteen times a minute, using about one-tenth of his maximum lung capacity. He thinks about his breathing only when some extra physical exertion—running for a bus or climbing several flights of stairs, for example—forces him to breathe faster and deeper than usual or when nasal congestion makes breathing difficult.

But sometimes an anxious climacteric male, although he is not exercising harder than usual, becomes tensely aware of his own breathing—the pumping of the lungs, the inflow and outflow of air through the nostrils and larynx. He thinks, "I need more air!" and consciously speeds up and deepens his breathing. It doesn't help: He can't seem to take in enough air; he feels that he is suffocating. Probably, at this stage, he also feels more or less severe palpitations; maybe he thinks he is having a heart attack.

In this desperate hunger for air, the terrified man may hyperventilate; he overbreathes—far beyond his normal requirements —to the point at which he blows off all the carbon dioxide from his system and shifts the blood from its usual slightly acid condition to alkalinity (respiratory alkalosis). Then he goes into tetany (in some ways resembling the symptoms produced by tetanus, or lockjaw): His face is contorted and his hands are clenched; he may become nearly unconscious.

Such an attack, fortunately, is self-limiting: After he exhausts himself, the patient automatically stops overbreathing and recovers. But he may still repeat the performance again and again until his neurosis is, for the time being, appeased.

This is the extreme form of air hunger. In milder forms this "respiratory neurosis" may manifest itself only in attacks of heavy sighing. Here the climacteric man is expressing in body language his dissatisfaction with, and his fear of, the life he is leading.

Some people mistake air hunger for shortness of breath; but shortness of breath is always caused either by physical exertion or by an ailment of the heart or lungs. Shortness of breath is accompanied by puffing or panting, which can be noticed by observers. Air hunger, however, is a subjective feeling. An attack can begin while a man is sitting quietly in a chair and can develop, unnoticed by onlookers, until it advances to the stage of hyperventilation.

Liver Spots

Liver spots have nothing to do with any disease of the liver. They are produced in white males by an abnormality of skin pigment and are so named because some of them resemble the color of cooked liver (although in different men, and even in different places on the same man, the spots may show various shades of dark brown and red-brown). They are not the same as freckles;

they are often darker than freckles, are not produced by exposure to sunlight, and may appear on men whose skin never freckled. They are not the same as moles; moles are usually present from childhood, are slightly raised, and sometimes are hairy. Liver spots appear in middle life, are flush with the skin surface, and are never hairy.

Most liver spots are covered by the clothing. However, big, dark liver spots on the hands or face may be quite conspicuous, and the man may become unduly conscious of them, seeing them as ominous signs that he is aging.

Headaches

Brain tissue itself is apparently insensitive to pain, but a number of other tissues of the head are quite sensitive. These include:

1. The meninges (men'-in-jeez), three membranes enclosing the brain;
2. The veins and arteries of the head, inside and outside the skull;
3. The fifth, ninth, and tenth cranial nerves;
4. The first three nerve roots from the cervical spinal cord (the neck part of the spinal cord);
5. The muscles of the neck and scalp.

All these tissues are sensitive to pain, and pain in any of them is called "headache." The headaches characteristic of the climacteric are usually produced by hormonal disturbances, stress, or emotional tension on the veins and arteries, cranial nerves, and muscles.

Dizziness

The man feels as if he were about to lose his balance; sometimes this dizziness is accompanied by a sensation of faintness.

It is much like the faint, dizzy feeling that some people experience when they quickly stand up after having been sitting or lying down for some time, but it is not necessarily produced by any such sudden movement. It can come on when a man is sitting still or when he is walking. In some cases there is vertigo—that is, a sensation of spinning around or of rocking, as in a boat on a rough sea.

Sometimes the total effect is mild. The man makes a slight conscious effort to do what is normally an unconscious process—maintaining his balance—and nobody else can detect what he is feeling. In other cases the dizziness and faintness are quite severe: The man comes close to losing consciousness; he has to stop whatever he is doing and may have to cling to something solid to stop himself from falling down. Dizziness in the climacteric male is usually a vasomotor effect—that is, caused by some disturbance of the blood flow, similar to those that cause hot flashes.

Osteoporosis

In osteoporosis (os-tee-ō-por-o-sis), derived from the Greek words *osteon* (bone) and *poros* (passage), the bones become more porous than they should be. Osteoporosis is not uncommon in advancing years (usually in the late fifties or sixties) and is found more frequently in women than in men. Backaches are common in this condition, often aggravated by collapse of one or more of the brittle vertebrae. Also, there is usually a greater susceptibility to fractures.

MENTAL AND EMOTIONAL SYMPTOMS

The symptoms described so far may be distressing to the climacteric man and his wife; yet most of them can easily be concealed from outsiders. The next group of symptoms are quite conspicuous; they will be obvious to the man's friends and fellow workers, yet, in some instances he himself will be the only one who is unaware of them.

Irritability

The man's temperament may change noticeably. He may become rude, short-tempered, impatient with his wife and children —in some instances physically cruel to them.

One woman described how, in several families she knew, the husband-wife relationship had deteriorated: "She became fearful of his attitude in many instances, and could not understand this *new man*." A woman describes her husband's behavior: "Sadistic; violent spells; sudden bursts of temper; bad language; suspicious, selfish, insensitive. He never felt there was anything wrong with him—only everybody else, particularly me." A man says of himself that his behavior became "very erratic; impatient; more emotional —almost in the extreme at times. Sometimes I was completely unreasonable, yet not morose about this afterwards, as I would have been in the past." Another man describes his brother-in-law:

> Is negative, suspicious, hostile toward society. Rants about how "the world is full of hatred." Violently criticizes politicians, teachers, all minorities, hippies, etc. Very self-centered. . . . Family and friends are always on edge around him, because no matter how sociable the occasion, and how normal and happy he seems, the wrong subject can set him off into fanatical raving. At one time he said, "Everyone I know is angry about the condition of the world. I know I'm always just boiling inside." Actually everyone *I* know doesn't feel that way, but he gravitates to people that share his attitudes. This man has three brothers, all over 50, who haven't shown any abnormal changes so far. His wife is concerned about him. She has psoriasis—no wonder!

Fatigue

The man begins to feel abnormally fatigued—more so than could be explained by his energy output at work or play or by the normal slight decline of strength associated with his increasing age. "Reduced drive at work," "Loss of energy and interest" are typical descriptions of the condition. Falling testosterone levels are often involved with such loss of stamina.

Insomnia

For some of the men who feel so tired so much of the day, nighttime brings no relief. They complain of lying awake for hours after going to bed, of restless sleep, of nightmares, or of waking several hours before it is time to get up in ·the morning.

This sleeplessness is characteristic of a chronic depressive anxiety state affecting the middle-aged man. He brings occupational problems home from work and adds them to his domestic worries. At work he is constantly in a hurry, and away from it he is constantly busy with family, in-laws, friends and neighbors, or meetings. He never finds time in his waking hours to sit down with a colleague, or with a member of his family, to talk out his problems; he never finds time to go for a walk by himself or just to sit still and think about his troubles. So they follow him to bed and haunt him when he seeks his badly needed rest. His overactive brain has found no time for contemplation during his waking hours, so it works overtime at night.

There is reason to believe that, during the rapid eye movement (REM) stage of sleep, the human brain sorts out and classifies the previous day's experiences, like a good filing clerk who clears the desk, ready for the next day. The insomniac does not properly accomplish this mental clearance during the night; when he awakes, he does not feel refreshed because the previous day's problems are still lingering on. So he is already fatigued, even before he begins the new day.

Moodiness and Depression

The most common type of depression is called exogenous depression, meaning that it is produced by outside causes. Middle-aged men are likely to have various distressing experiences—death of a wife, financial loss, forced retirement from well-liked employment, and so on.

The man feels sad, he loses interest in things and people he formerly enjoyed; he becomes sluggish and inactive. He develops a low opinion of himself and perhaps begins to neglect his clothing and bodily cleanliness. He feels that things are never going to improve.

Said one man: "It's very difficult to be optimistic about the future, with everything being on the downgrade." William K., who in reality is no worse off than most other middle-aged men, feels constantly depressed by the thought that his life savings, and the retirement fund that he worked so hard to accumulate, could be devalued or could even disappear completely, leaving him a pauper in his old age.

Another type of depression is called endogenous depression (sometimes called psychotic depression) and has no discernible outside cause but arises from within the man's own personality. One man described it well: "Depression; lack of confidence in my own abilities and others; sense of futility with life; a strong cynicism combined with a strong restlessness; generally a strong feeling of dissatisfaction with my life and the way I was living, although I could not determine what I was actually dissatisfied with."

Endogenous depression is considered the more serious of the two forms. Some cases may include a break with reality—for example, unrealistic notions of self-worthlessness or delusions of being persecuted. One man complained, "It seems at times as if there was a plot against me. Everybody is out to get me." Another man developed a sudden interest in religion. He said, "All those years I thought I knew what I was meant to do and to be, but it's only lately that I discovered my true calling; I am meant to be a prophet, a guru, a leader of the people in bondage and ignorance. Now I'm against the system I once believed in."

In severe cases of depression there may be attempts at suicide.

Weakened Mental Ability

The man's mental powers—memory, concentration, decisiveness, among others—become seriously weakened, partly due to aging, partly due to hormone fluctuations. A man said, "At work I run a big drill press. I happen to need something from my tool box; I walk over about fifty feet to where it is, and by the time I get there I've forgotten what I need. It's much the same away from work: If I have several things to do, I'll often forget the most important item."

Some men, formerly alert, decisive, and active, become absent-minded, careless, and procrastinating. Tasks that used to be easy become tiresome.

Some men lose interest in their own affairs and in other people: They become bored and apathetic. A man says that he developed "indifference to the point where a conscious mental effort was required for even the most minor out-of-routine tasks."

Loss of Self-Confidence

One might expect that a man, as he reached middle age, would become more self-confident. He has overcome the shyness and fears of youth and knows how to deal with women and with other men. He is experienced in his work; he has learned how to handle his own financial affairs. Yet many men at the climacteric suddenly lose this well-established self-confidence: They feel nervous, apprehensive, insecure.

A nurse reported, with regard to a patient, that he had "become uncertain of self—frightened—mildly schizophrenic." A woman said that her husband "could no longer indulge in arguments without becoming extremely nervous." A man, describing his own experiences, mentioned "doubt about virility and the need to demonstrate its unimpaired presence. . . . Awareness of economic vulnerability, especially during the last few years when promotion might be slow."

Behavior Changes

By the time a man reaches middle age, his life is regulated largely by habit. His manner of speech, his style of dress, his hair style, his tastes in food and drink, his method of handling money, his spare-time activities—all these are firmly established. His family and friends think that they know him fairly well. Yet sometimes you see a man suddenly diverge from his well-established life-style into a mode of behavior that seems inappropriate, even ridiculous.

One man, referring to himself and some of his friends, mentions "purchase of flashy cars; attempts to participate in new, unsuitable sports—skiing, perhaps." A woman observes in her husband and male friends "a 'youth reversion': youthful-style clothes and vocabulary; a faster car; extra attention to appearance (concern about baldness). In general, a desire to be a swinger, to recapture youth."

There may be a radical change in his attitude to life. A man says, "The most profound change was toward work. I realized that perhaps my entire past business career was simply a waste of time. This resulted in my attitude to the growth ethic and 'selling' of competitive free enterprise being changed. I began to research and write a book about the subject, but as I researched the angrier I became and the more critical the book became. . . ."

A woman said that at about the age of forty-five, her husband showed several changes of behavior: "Less inclined to have visitors in the home; authoritarian to [adult] children and spouse; more enthusiasm for male friends; inclination to purchase 'mod' clothes."

Age at Onset of Symptoms

One cannot be dogmatic about the age at which the climacteric begins. Many cases are not reported until long after the symptoms begin; many other cases are never reported at all (in the sense of being presented to a doctor for diagnosis and treatment). I would say, roughly, that of the cases that have come to my attention, three-quarters began between the ages of forty-one and fifty, the remainder between fifty-one and sixty.

PERIODICITY

Some of the symptoms described above are characteristically intermittent—for example, hot flashes, air hunger, headaches, memory lapses, dizziness, loss of self-confidence and depressive phases, diminished sexual potency. In some men it appears that such symptoms come and go irregularly; other men report a definite periodicity to their symptoms. A whole group of symptoms will come on together and last for awhile (usually a few days); then they will all vanish, and the man will be free of them for a time.

In one case the symptoms recurred every second or third day; in another the time was three or four weeks. For one man the main spells of symptoms recurred about every forty days, but there were often short spells in between. In another case there were intervals of six months to a year between spells.

One woman reported that for her exhusband, the physical symptoms remained constant; but his emotional symptoms—withdrawal, moodiness, and irritability—came and went on an approximate monthly cycle.

WARNING

I must emphasize that many of the symptoms described in this chapter can be caused not only by the climacteric but also by various diseases. Some such diseases are mentioned in Chapter 7. The man who experiences such symptoms, then, should not shrug them off as "just the climacteric"; he should get professional advice to find out for certain what is causing them.

2
Sex and Family Life

A man may easily be several months, or even years, into the climacteric and not realize what is the matter with him. There are several reasons, the first and most obvious of which is that he may never have heard of the male climacteric. Until recently it was discussed in only a few books and magazine articles.

Second, the syndrome varies markedly from one man to another; one man may give up all sexual activity, for example, while another is frantically chasing young women. (I would emphasize, by the way, the word "syndrome": The climacteric produces a *group* of symptoms. Some of them are part of the ordinary aging process; some are ill-defined sociological and psychosomatic symptoms; and some are not apparent to anyone but the man himself.)

Third, although in a minority of cases certain symptoms may come on suddenly, for most men there is no sudden, definite onset. With influenza, for example, a man knows that one day he feels all right and the next day he is sick. It is usually not so with the climacteric.

Fourth, further confusing the situation is the fact that for some men symptoms may be intermittent. If the spells of symptoms recur at fairly long, irregular intervals, a man may not perceive them as manifestations of the one underlying condition: He may simply think he is suffering a series of disconnected illnesses.

SUFFERING IN SILENCE

I want to discuss first the man's own reaction to the climacteric, because in most cases it differs markedly from a wife's reaction.

We do not know exactly how many men at the climacteric suffer loss of potency or of libido. Some such cases are reported to the physician or psychiatrist, but many are not. Some men are embarrassed to go; even the hope of regaining their vanishing virility will not overcome their reluctance to discuss it with the doctor.

It is not the sort of thing, either, that the average man admits to his friends. Any form of male sexual inadequacy is, in our society, considered a fit subject for ridicule (although frigidity in a woman is not). So, from boyhood the male learns to brag about his prowess—truthfully if he can, falsely if he must. He hears his friends similarly boasting about their potency; he cannot know whether they are lying, so he assumes that they are speaking the truth.

Most men will accept the fact that as they grow older, their physical strength gradually declines: At forty-five one cannot swim, play golf, or dance as long or as vigorously as one could at twenty-five. Yet many men don't like to accept the gradual decline of sexuality that, as I said in Chapter 1, normally accompanies aging.

I hope this book will help men to take a less emotional, more reasonable view of their sex lives. Then they will be able to quit the bragging. Then, too, as they grow older, they will be able to accept their declining sexuality without fear or shame, and to discuss it with their friends, doctors or wives as frankly as they now speak of graying hair or diminishing muscular strength. (Sex education will help, too, if it is true sex *education* and not simply a course in the biology of reproduction.)

Age and Sexuality

I would emphasize that under favorable conditions the decline in sexuality is only *gradual*. (By "favorable conditions" I mean the availability of a sex partner and fairly good general health.)

Men in their mid-twenties on the average have about three sex acts a week; by the mid-forties the average frequency is two; by the late fifties, one. As a compensation, many middle-aged men find that the contact of penis with vagina and the short, intense thrill of orgasm are no longer the predominant ingredients of the sex act: A wide range of emotional, verbal, and physical stimuli can be used to obtain a much-prolonged, exquisitely pleasurable experience.

Some men find in all this a change for the better. Nevertheless, many men don't like to accept a decline in sexuality.

Still less are they ready to accept the severe impairment of the sex life that so often occurs at the climacteric.

Sexuality and Secrecy

The man whose sexual powers are failing has seldom or never heard anyone else admit to the same problem. So he thinks that his own case is exceptional, and his feeling of shame is confirmed and deepened.

The nineteenth-century makers of Man Medicine cleverly took advantage of this masculine shame. They advertised that the Man Medicine formula would be given, free of charge, to any man who wrote for it. The impotent man received the formula easily enough but found that he could not concoct it himself; it would have to be made up by a pharmacist. He was ashamed to take it to the local drugstore, where everyone knew him, so he accepted the manufacturer's alternative offer to supply the ready-made medicine by mail.

Physicians are often unaware of their male patients' sexual problems. Many doctors do not specifically ask about this subject when making examinations. Even if the doctor does ask, many men will lie; and because there is no medical test to diagnose impotence, the doctor has to accept the patient's word. One man said that he sought no medical treatment for the climacteric "because, like a fever, once one has it one might just as well ride it out, and in the process build up antibodies which tend to give immunity from further attacks."

Another man, asked if he had taken any treatment, replied, "Not yet. I hadn't considered the problem to be this serious, and felt I was helping my worst problems with positive attitude." (A positive attitude will not work in every case. It cannot relieve problems that are not at the conscious level: These have to be brought up into consciousness before they can be dealt with.)

Many men whose sexuality is flagging will even try to conceal it from wives. Here are some of the methods they may use:

1. The tired businessman method: The man complains that he is much busier at work than he used to be. Perhaps he comes home very late. Anyway, whatever time he does get in, he is too tired for sex.

2. The television addict approach: The man develops an overpowering interest in late-night shows. By the time he comes to bed, his wife is asleep; or if she is not, he can reasonably say that it is too late for sex.

3. The "I-can't-be-bothered" syndrome: The man has periods of emotional coolness when he doesn't want to be approached or touched by his wife. Such a period may come on immediately after one completed act of intercourse (or after an unsuccessful attempt) and may last two weeks or more.

4. The not-speaking tactic: The man picks a quarrel with his wife. He begins to criticize the way she is bringing up the kids; he finds fault with her handling of the family budget; or he complains that she neglects to cook his favorite dinner recipes. Anyway, on whatever pretext, they fight. He sulks; and then, when you're not on speaking terms with a woman, how can you make love to her? The alienation can be continued until (if ever) the man feels up to another attempt at sexual activity.

These methods may not be consciously planned. For most men, assurance of their own virility is a basic need, and many have accepted the fallacy that "potency on demand" is the one measure of manliness. Therefore many men unconsciously find ways to avoid facing up to the diminution or loss of such narrowly conceived "manliness."

Anyway, whether it is consciously or unconsciously practiced, the purpose of deception is to avoid the threat of scorn or rejection that the man fears, were he to be frank with his wife. (If one of these men did manage to bring the problem into the open, he would quite likely find, to his surprise, that the wife is not nearly so worried about the record of sexual performance as he is and would not dream of scoffing at him or rejecting him.)

No Secret

Whether a man speaks about his symptoms or not, a wife knows that something is the matter with him. How can she not notice it if he begins applying the tactics described above or if he keeps himself busy every night with reading, handicrafts, or work until she has gone to sleep? In this way he escapes the embarrassment of sexual failure in bed; yet the wife can deduce that he has lost his libido or has become impotent. Alternatively, his failure to communicate may lead her to suspect that her husband has a lover and is spending all his sexual powers on the other woman.

Nonsexual symptoms, too, will be noticed by the wife. If the man who used to sleep well spends hours each night tossing and turning in the dark or switches on the bed-lamp to read, the wife knows. She notices the urine-soiled shorts of the prostate sufferer. If he develops liver spots on his hands or body, his wife will see them. If he suffers from itching and formication, even though he does not complain, his wife will see him scratching.

Lapses of memory cannot always be concealed. A widow, asked about her late husband, said, "He had lapses of memory. . . . At times I would mention things to him; if I brought it up again he would not remember them. I'd say, 'But, Tommy, I told you this!' He'd say, 'No, I don't remember you telling me that.' This was getting to be more frequent."

In some cases, although the wife realizes that the husband is not his old self, she dare not talk to him about it. One woman said, "He believes that a male climacteric is a myth—mentioning it is the red flag to a bull!" Such a breakdown of communications may have unpleasant results for the woman: Because of the strains associated with the menopause, she may urgently need ego support, yet her husband does not give it. (I'm not blaming the husband: His own ego may be just as shaky as hers.)

THE APHRODITE COMPLEX

An old Greek legend tells how Zeus, king of the gods, fell in love with his own daughter, Aphrodite, and gave her a child, who turned out to be Eros, the little god of love. From this legend I have taken a name for the phenomenon, quite common in the climacteric, of men chasing women young enough to be their own daughters.

A man has noticed his sexual powers declining and thinks, "It's only because my wife is aging. When she was better looking, I was virile enough! What I need, to get back my lost manhood, is a younger, prettier woman." So off he goes and finds one. The results may not be satisfactory.

One man, describing his own experiences, writes, "The change began between forty and fifty . . . doubt about virility and the need to demonstrate its unimpaired presence; frequent disastrous involvements with younger women, where the authority of age and position is used as a power play. Panic when affairs became too serious." This panic reaction is by no means uncommon.

Charles Dickens, in his mid-forties, moved into a separate bedroom from Catherine, his wife, and took as his mistress an actress named Ellen Ternan, nineteen years old. He actually ordered his wife to pay a formal visit to his mistress. To the dismay of friends and the astonishment of readers, he printed in the June 12, 1858, edition of his magazine *Household Words* a front-page story about his separation from Catherine. Dickens had been an exceptionally active, athletic man; but by the time he was going through this sexual upheaval, he wrote to Wilkie Collins, "I am not quite well —can't get quite well."

When H. G. Wells was forty-six, he began to show uncharacteristic aggressiveness and bad temper; he experienced alternate moods of elation and depression. And he struck up a love affair with a woman aged twenty.

Sometimes the man will be absurdly ostentatious in the conduct of his extramarital affair. For some such men, it is an ego-boost to be seen around town with a glamorous young woman. Other men—with an exaggerated sense of righteousness—may feel unconsciously guilty, to the point where they want to be caught cheating, in order to be properly penalized for their offense.

The man who can maintain a satisfactory, long-lasting relationship with a young woman has, from his point of view, solved the problem of his flagging sexuality. Yet, for many men the attempt does not succeed.

A man already feels inadequate and embarrassed if he has failed sexually with his wife. He begins to fear that he may fail again with the new woman; this fear increases the likelihood of failure. Now, if he does indeed fail, he feels worse than before: By that failure he has demolished his old excuse—his wife's fading charms—and has to admit his own responsibility.

And if his performance in bed with the new woman is below expectations, the man may not be able to find much consolation out of bed. In their search for women, many middle-aged men are initially attracted by youth and sex appeal; they do not bother looking for integrated personality, brains, or conversational ability. The man feels embarrassed, and the young woman may very well feel bored. One middle-aged man described "the end of an extra-curricular affair, an unkind remark by a young thing regarding advancing years, etc." In many cases the man is not satisfied with an extramarital affair and marries the younger woman. Yet the second honeymoon cannot ensure his sexual revitalization.

Another man summed up his experience as "Sexual withdrawal . . . divorce, several hopeless relationships with women."

So the transfer of sexual attentions to a younger woman (with or without divorce) is by no means a sure cure for the middle-aged man's flagging sexuality.

The following is a case that exemplifies several of the points mentioned above.

Len, a handsome and superficially charming man of forty-eight, was comfortably settled with a middle-aged wife, Margery, and four growing children. But Len got bored with Margery and decided to leave home and seek adventure elsewhere.

He began to see a lot of a twenty-six-year-old divorcée, Anne, who lived quite near his former home. The kids wondered why Daddy's car was so often parked close by and yet Daddy was not living at home now. Margery had to conjure up some fancy stories to keep them quiet.

Len had left his family without financial support, so they were living on welfare. Yet he occasionally came to visit them, bringing gifts for all the kids. For Margery, these visits were agonizing. He bullied her, warning her not to get involved with other men; he criticized her efforts as homemaker and mother; he sneered at her peptic ulcer and her migraine as being all hypochondria, ignoring his own role in causing these ailments.

After awhile Len moved in with Anne, expecting to enjoy all the sex and excitement he felt he was entitled to. But he was unable to fulfill her expectations for sex, dancing, drinking, and swinging. Eventually she threw him out.

I have discussed the situation in which the climacteric man makes up his mind that he needs a younger woman. Yet sometimes a man who would not have thought of such a thing himself has the idea put into his head by a woman.

Suppose the man's loss of libido makes his wife suspicious: She accuses him of having a girl friend and of squandering away from home all the potency he ought to be saving for use at home. The man thinks, "I'm already condemned, so why shouldn't I have the pleasure of committing the crime?" Or perhaps, just when he is emotionally upset by the climacteric, a man meets a young woman who, for one reason or another, feels strongly attracted to older men. The following is an instance that shows how easily this can happen.

A climacteric psychiatrist, aged fifty, has a neurotic female patient of thirty-one. For more than a year she faithfully attends interviews and counseling sessions with him, finding them increasingly enjoyable. She feels secure in the sanctity of the doctor's office and comforted by the genuine care that he projects. She feels strongly attracted by this wise, impressive father-figure and eventually falls in love with him. She has never loved anyone like this before and becomes flirtatious to the point of seductiveness. She is good-looking and intelligent; the psychiatrist is strongly tempted to get sexually involved with her.

In this particular case the affair was not consummated. The psychiatrist, through fear of professional disgrace (and also through fear that he might be impotent with her) backed away. At the last minute the woman panicked, too, because she did not really want a sexual involvement. Her feeling for him turned to dislike, and she transferred to another psychiatrist.

Many middle-aged men, less cautious than this psychiatrist, are tempted by the advances of younger women. (The relationship between obstetrician and patient, for example, is often mistaken, by one or both of them, for sexual love.) The results are seldom wholly satisfactory. One reason is that most women who fall in love with, or marry, men twenty years or more older than themselves are emotionally of a particular personality type. The average young woman desires a man who will be her lover and husband and father to her children; but it may well be that the woman who falls in love with and marries a much older man subconsciously desires someone who will serve as father to her. With this motivation, how long can she be happy in the role of wife?

TALKING IT OVER

I have described a number of cases in which the husband and wife cannot freely talk about the physical and emotional problems associated with the climacteric. There are, of course, many couples who can discuss the subject without embarrassment.

A widow said, concerning her late husband, "I recall very well when he couldn't make love. I was concerned, not for myself, but for him. I even suggested that he go elsewhere—you know, find someone and pay them; but he said, 'No, dear; that's why I married you.' He maintained this right to the day he died."

I don't know how many wives make such suggestions, but there's no doubt that, with or without wifely permission, many husbands follow this advice. Call girls and "massage parlors" are patronized less by single men than by middle-aged, middle-class married men, who are charged accordingly. For some men the prostitute plays another role besides that of providing sex: She may serve as a sympathetic listener, a sort of mother-confessor. Such men can talk more frankly to prostitutes than they ever would to their wives.

The wife may persuade her husband to see a doctor. Yet sometimes that produces no great improvement. Several men report undergoing medical examinations and being told that nothing was wrong. The man perhaps has not been frank with the physician. He may complain about being "run down" or of having indigestion or insomnia but may not mention the symptoms that are bothering him (and his wife) the most.

Many men refuse to get medical advice. Nowadays, indeed, it is often the wife who visits a doctor to complain about, and seek a cure for, her husband's lost sex drive. Yet some wives, too, would be embarrassed to see a doctor—particularly a male doctor—on such a matter, and so they say nothing.

Unfortunately, talking it over does not always solve the problem. Mrs. B., a real-estate saleswoman of forty-four, had a husband of forty-eight; they were happy with their marriage and their sixteen-year-old daughter. Mr. B. began to make occasional remarks about being bored with their life together; he spoke wistfully of the fun he had missed by marrying too young. Mrs. B. did not take his complaints seriously, even when he went on to hint at a temporary separation. She did not intend to move out herself; neither would she ask him to leave. For eighteen months they talked from time to time about Mr. B.'s dissatisfaction, but the wife never felt particularly worried. It was just a phase, she thought: He would get over it.

He did not get over it. One day he told her he was through; he still respected her, but she no longer turned him on physically. She could keep the house and furnishings, he said; she could keep the daughter (now eighteen years old), and he would pay half the cost of supporting her. He voluntarily took all the blame himself and gave her no time for discussion. His bags were already packed; he picked them up and walked out.

He moved into an apartment, outfitted himself with mod, youthful clothes, let his hair grow long and dyed it red, bought a flashy new automobile, and began to live it up with the girls. Mrs. B. just could not understand such a radical character change in a formerly responsible, reliable, loving husband. She panicked and before long was hospitalized in a state of acute depressive anxiety.

She had never before heard of the male climacteric, so it was explained to her. She now realizes that she was not to blame for the disintegration of their marriage. She knows that Mr. B. may, sooner or later, come to his senses; but she feels that his pride would not let him come back for a reconciliation after having gone so far.

GOOD RIDDANCE!

For some couples the loss or sharp reduction of the man's sexuality will not produce much emotional upheaval: Their sex life is already unsatisfactory. I said earlier that many men are secretive about their sexuality right through their adult lives. I believe that many men and woman similarly hide the fact that they have found sex life in marriage bitterly disappointing. The following are some common cases for such disappointment.

Boredom

Many couples get bored with sex. They do not know that it is possible, or will not take the trouble, to maintain a spirit of courtship or to use a variety of erotic techniques. Sexual boredom is more likely among working-class than middle-class couples because sex plays a bigger part in working-class lives. Middle-class people tend to sublimate some of their sex drive into other activities and consequently do not get bored so easily with it.

Sex As a Weapon

A wife may have developed the technique of punishing her husband by refusing sexual relations when he wants them. This tactic, repeated often enough, can destroy the husband's interest in her; their sex life has come to an end long before he begins to feel the effects of the climacteric.

The Disappointed Wife

Many a man loves his wife, yet demonstrates that love only by intercourse—no loving words, caresses, or gifts. The wife eventually comes to think, "That's all he wants me for!" Her enthusiasm for intercourse declines, and she finds excuses for avoiding it. She may not much care when he loses the ability to provide it.

The Inadequate Husband

Some husbands, right from the wedding day, are sexually inadequate. So when such a man experiences the climacteric, his wife may feel she has not lost much anyway. "Perhaps he would have benefited from hormone treatment," says one wife of her husband, "but middle age only accentuated his lack of sexual capability."

The Frigid Wife

There are many wives who, for physical or emotional reasons, find sex repugnant. Soon after the wedding the man realizes that his wife dislikes his lovemaking. Perhaps she put on a good act during courtship; later she admits the truth—perhaps only to herself, perhaps to her husband as well.

Some such women get deeply involved in outside activities—social, philanthropic, religious, political, and so on—that keep them away from home for much of the time and absorb much of their physical and emotional energy. (This is the housewife's equivalent of the "tired businessman strategy" that I described earlier in this chapter.) It reduces the time available for sexual activity at home; in many cases, it is destructive to the husband's ego because it makes him feel rejected.

Undoubtedly, the frigid wife will not be worried much if the male climacteric deprives her of her husband's sexual attentions: Far from complaining, she may keep her fingers crossed and hope he never recovers.

LOVING AND MAKING LOVE

Many men at the climacteric lose their ability, or their desire, to "make love" in the physical sense. Yet a more serious problem, as far as many women are concerned, arises when the husband loses his ability, or forgets how, to "love" in the emotional sense—to care for his wife and to *show* his affection warmly, expressively, and frequently. Women are more likely to feel threatened by such an emotional failure than by the man's failure to achieve and maintain an erection.

One woman described her reaction to this lack of emotional love: "I felt very much ignored, not needed. The fact that the growing children did not need me any more was hard to accept. On top of that, it seemed that my husband did not need me, either.

For a time I left him alone completely; now he realizes that he still needs a companion. A woman must try very hard to be patient and understanding."

How Many?

I would say that loss of potency or libido is much more common than is generally supposed; and it is not a new phenomenon. Here is a suggestive fact: In 1914, when there were about eight million men between forty and sixty years of age in the United States, *one* of the many "lost-manhood" patent-medicine firms had a mailing list of half a million names! Lost manhood was obviously big business.

Family Life

For many families the sharpest parent-child conflicts occur when the children are in their teens. This situation is difficult enough when parents can bring to it their best endowment of understanding, tolerance, and love; it will be much more difficult if at the same time the father, in his late forties or early fifties, is going through the male climacteric.

If the father is suffering from frequent headaches, he is likely to complain about the noise the children make. If he exhibits sudden changes of behavior—uncharacteristic, inappropriate ways of dressing, talking, acting—he may embarrass his family.

Irritability, moodiness, depression, delusions—all these may make life unpleasant for a man's wife and family. One woman says that her husband

wanted to be alone; isolated himself and his wife from the world. He withdrew from the world and lay on the sofa from Friday to Monday. He accused me of infidelity, said I was never home, though I was there seven days a week.

Though we had always had a joint account, I rarely used it. I spent my own earnings on the household, myself, and our daughter. Now he accused me of constantly taking his money and wanted *all* the money in his name.

He got suspicious of his food, accused me of being a mental case and of trying to kill him. He adopted the attitude that he was okay but I was a real monster.

I know several men who had been gentle all their life; they turned into real despots. One would accept no phone calls or let anyone else call out.

The children are not directly concerned with the sexual symptoms of the climacteric (except in those cases where the man falls in love with his own daughter); yet they will obviously be affected by sex-based misunderstandings and quarrels between the parents. I saw an installment of the TV series "Marcus Welby, M.D." that dealt with this problem. A middle-aged man who had become impotent with his wife took a young mistress in hopes of rejuvenating himself. He excused his evening absences from home by saying that he was attending psychotherapy sessions. One evening he was in a restaurant, having dinner with his mistress, when in walked his teen-age daughter with her boyfriend and caught her father and his young love holding hands.

The daughter, who had worshipped her father, was now involved in a severe love-hate conflict. She suffered such a bad attack of asthma that she had to be hospitalized. Every time her father visited her, the asthma grew worse because she could not express to him her hatred of what she saw as his hypocrisy.

Eventually the doctor discovered the cause of the trouble. He helped the daughter to recognize the climacteric crisis that her father was undergoing. When she understood the situation, she was able to vent her feelings and relieve the pressure of the love-hate conflict. Once that was done, she soon recovered and could feel compassion for her father's problem.

Not all children are lucky enough to get such sound advice. Thus, for many of them the father's change of character and behavior and the consequent disruption of formerly happy father-child relationships may cause long-lasting physical or emotional damage. The children will also suffer if, through weakened mental ability or other emotional symptoms, their father loses his job, starts making foolish investments, gambles, or otherwise gets into economic difficulties.

Fathers, on the other hand, may suffer because of their children's inability to understand the physical and mental problems of middle age. One man, feeling the symptoms of the climacteric, was not helped by his daughter's remark, "But Daddy, at your age you're almost dead already!"

THE SINGLE MAN

So far I have dealt in this chapter with married men; yet the climacteric may affect bachelors, widowers, and divorced and separated men as well. If the man has not enjoyed an active sex life, then the sexual symptoms of the climacteric will have little effect on him. It may, indeed, prove helpful if he stops craving for the sexual pleasures that, for some reason or other, he is not getting. If he has been satisfying himself by masturbation, he may simply lose the desire to do it; it may be somewhat frustrating if he retains the desire but loses the ability.

The man's friends may notice some of the nonsexual symptoms. A divorced woman in her mid-forties was friendly with a divorced man a few years older. One Sunday they were to take a hike in the country. She reports, "That morning when he arrived to pick me up, he said, 'I'm not satisfied with the name your parents gave you; from now on, I'm going to call you Cecile.' All that day he did call me Cecile; but, next time we met, he used my proper name and never mentioned the Cecile idea again."

What had probably happened was that the man had forgotten her real name and had invented the "Cecile" fiction to conceal his lapse. The ruse succeeded with this woman, who did not know him very well (although, of course, it puzzled her); it might not have worked with a wife or lover.

THE CLIMACTERIC AND THE MENOPAUSE

The male climacteric results from a physiological and hormonal aging process, usually complicated by various psychological and social problems. The same general terms could be used to describe the menopause.

Many men fail to understand the woman's problems with the menopause; many women fail to understand the man's problems with the climacteric. So in this chapter it may be helpful to mention some of the differences between the two conditions and the different ways in which women and men react to them:

1. The menopause is inevitable; the male climacteric is uncertain, and many men never experience it at all.

2. The woman expects the menopause, is emotionally prepared for it, and can easily get advice from friends, books, or physicians on how to cope with it. The typical man is not prepared for the climacteric; when it comes, he does not know what is happening to him and may not get any useful advice.

3. For some men the climacteric severely curtails their sexual ability; the menopause does not have the same effect on women, although their libido may be reduced.

4. The man in midlife has about six years less life expectancy (that is, a greater risk of early death) than a woman of the same age. (In Chapter 6 I give some statistics to demonstrate this fact.) To men who are aware of their shorter life expectancy, signs of physical deterioration may seem more threatening than they do to women.

5. In most men the awareness of aging seems to strike more unexpectedly than in women. The man who had always seen himself as being young and vigorous all at once begins to think of disease, decrepitude, and death. For a man who is emotionally

vulnerable, this disintegration of the self-image will enhance the development of the climacteric syndrome.

It is fair to say, then, that even for a man who is prepared for it, the climacteric is at least as emotionally disturbing as the menopause is for a woman; for the many men who are not prepared for it, it may be more so.

3
The Man in Society

For many men work is the most important thing in their lives—more important than their wives (how often one hears this complaint from wives!), more important than children, hobbies, religion, or politics. A married man who is so work-obsessed may not worry if at the climacteric he loses his libido. Quite likely, through lack of time and physical exhaustion, he may have only rarely made love to his wife anyway in recent years, so he may feel he is not missing much.

This long-term work obsession is different from the tired-businessman method described earlier. But the truly work-obsessed man—let him suddenly find that he cannot work so hard or so well as he once could—let him find his status diminished among colleagues or competitors—let him feel his security threatened—*then* he is deeply concerned.

THE EMPLOYEE

Such symptoms as lapses of memory, inability to concentrate, chronic fatigue and headaches reduce a man's efficiency at work. Moodiness, spells of depression and irritability impair his relations with fellow workers. If he has to deal with the public, these same emotional symptoms make that aspect of his work more irritating than before.

"I tended to suffer fools less," says one man, "had a feeling of cool determination, but while trying to maintain civility, was more outspoken, less long-suffering." Another man described his "awareness of economic vulnerability, especially during the last few years when promotions might be slow, although income may be higher than ever."

The man may worry about younger men nipping at his heels; he may feel aggrieved that other people don't understand all his difficulties; he may receive pity from those who do partly understand, which in turn lowers his already shaken self-esteem.

Some men react differently; they cannot see anything wrong with themselves at all. There is a significant parallel here with a situation I described in Chapter 2. It often happens that the man whose sexual powers fail will blame his wife for not being attractive enough to stimulate him. Similarly, the man who can't admit that his working powers are failing will begin to blame the job.

One man reported: "Perhaps my entire past business career was a waste of time. . . . I was quite literally shunned and avoided toward the end, and it was quite a relief to my boss when I finally quit, I'm sure." Another man mentioned "a dissatisfaction with present job, a lament for missed opportunities."

When the employee feels that his work is not worth doing anyway, that it is a "swindle," that it is beneath him, that he made a mistake in ever getting involved with it, then he can rationalize his own dwindling efficiency. "I *could* do better," he thinks, "but why the hell *should* I?" He becomes resentful, hard to deal with and unreliable. I suspect that many a saboteur inside business and industry is motivated by such a climacteric identity-crisis.

The following case illustrates how a man at the climacteric may create imaginary difficulties for himself and make life uncomfortable for his fellow workers. Doctor J. G., chief of staff of a 350-bed district hospital, was in his early fifties. He was competent and experienced, to be sure, yet he had an unrealistically high opinion of himself (probably an overcompensated inferiority complex); to protect it, he was as alert and savage as a watchdog. He ruled the house staff and resident doctors with an iron hand; behind his back they called him "the Chief"; and woe betide any of them who dared compete with the Chief in any way!

J. G. went on vacation, leaving one of his assistants in charge of his private patients. The young surgeon felt honored and tried his best to give good service, hoping to win some commendation when the Chief returned. Instead, he received a severe dressing-down for his pains:

> I suppose you're hoping to win my patients over from me! You seem to have the delusion that you can cover up a lack of medical skill and experience with personal charm and social graces. But you can't fool people very long like that, you know.
>
> Another thing: I notice that you've slowly but surely veered away from my established routine, introducing unorthodox, un-tested methods of your own! Just what are you trying to do: establish a new dynasty? How insubordinate can one get? Don't you know who's boss around here?

Irrational fear of aging, anxiety about loss of prestige and iden-tity, irrational jealousy of younger men, and panicky defense against nonexistent threats to one's livelihood—these are typical climacteric reactions in the ambitious man who has achieved some success.

THE EMPLOYER

An employer who begins to exhibit the emotional symptoms of the climacteric can become a terror to his staff—unpredictable, unfair, the most-hated man in the firm. He may be rash in his judgment of business affairs, slow to take necessary action, or wildly changeable in his decisions, as his moods alternate between the optimistic and pessimistic.

Some corporations recognize the risks to their employees—and hence to the employers themselves—of the midlife crisis. They systematically watch for the first signs of its onset. Two common indications are, first, when a man who had formerly done his work well suddenly begins to neglect it or to make a lot of mistakes and, second, when a man who had formerly got along well with fellow workers suddenly becomes excessively critical of them.

The prudent employer, detecting such signs of the climacteric in an employee, will take care that the man gets whatever treatment may be needed to restore him to good health and full productivity. Even if the employer bears part, or all, of the cost, it can be a good investment.

CLIMACTERIC CLIMBERS

The unpleasant effects of the climacteric as described above are seen principally among middle-class business and professional men, the sort of men who assume that they should continually advance in their careers, increasing their earnings as they grow older. Most manual workers, on the other hand, realize that their strength will decline and that they will be able to do less work as they grow older.

Some other societies—Mexico and India, for example—place less emphasis on competition and financial success than we do. There, fewer middle-aged men would worry about the physical and emotional effects of the climacteric. And when a man worries less about a situation, its effects automatically become less burdensome; symptoms are worsened by worry.

I have spoken so far about the problems of employees and employers. But the self-employed are not necessarily immune. A few historical cases suggest that the climacteric affects famous, highly accomplished men as readily as the laborer.

The life of Leo Tolstoy seems to show how the climacteric may upset the career of a writer. Tolstoy was born in 1828. In 1876, when he was about forty-eight years old, he suffered a frightening lapse of memory. He stepped out of his study one evening and suddenly forgot where he was—he could not recognize his own house. He had to call for help; his wife came and showed him the way to his bedroom. For the next few months, he suffered spells of severe depression, neglected his writing, and began to contemplate suicide. In the spring of 1877 he experienced a sudden religious conversion and became very devout.

Here was a complete transformation of character: The formerly prolific author had just about ceased to write; the former skeptic, who had for years bitterly attacked the Orthodox Church, now followed a routine of prayer, fasting, confession, and communion. (The sudden turn—or return—to religion is quite common among men of this age. I have often seen it in my own church.)

About the end of 1879 the climacteric (if that is what was influencing Tolstoy) passed off. He began eating meat on fasting days and renewed his spoken and written attacts on the church. He launched into a new period of vigorous literary creativity.

Born in 1564, William Shakespeare was for most of his career an extraordinarily prolific, successful playwright. Many people have thought it strange that he retired at what we should consider the early age of forty-six. Yet his writings yield clues that suggest that Shakespeare was a victim of the male climacteric. Two plays that he wrote in his early forties—*King Lear* (c. 1605) and *Timon of Athens* (c. 1608)—deal with middle-aged men who undergo sudden transformations of character that eventually wreck their lives.

Let us consider Lear's behavior as symptomatic of the climacteric. First, as king of Britain he suddenly announces that he is going to resign his crown and divide the kingdom among his three young daughters (a highly eccentric action in itself). His cantankerous behavior to Cordelia in Act I, Scene 1 would be unbelievable in a normal man: It is characteristic of a man at the climacteric. In the same scene he rages at his best advisor, Kent, and banishes him. Later in the same scene Goneril says, "You see how full of changes his age is." In Act I, Scene 3, Goneril tells Lear to "put away these dispositions that of late transform you from what you rightly are." A little later Lear bursts into tears!

Timon of Athens, a kindly, easygoing, generous man, suddenly undergoes a character transformation: He sees the world as full of baseness, selfishness, and ingratitude; he turns from his old philanthropy to a bitter hatred of all mankind. In Act V, Scene 1, the First Senator seems to imply that Timon's character change has a physical cause: "His discontents are unremovably coupled to nature."

Two plays that Shakespeare is known to have written after Timon—*Pericles, Prince of Tyre* (c. 1608), and *Henry VIII* (c. 1611)—are grossly inferior to his earlier work. He was not able to complete them by himself; his parts of the scripts were filled out to the required length by other writers.

There is some evidence that Shakespeare's sex life with his wife had ended before he was forty-five. So we may fairly ask whether Shakespeare quit the theater because the mental and emotional changes of the climacteric had so eroded his creative ability that he could not continue.

When the climacteric disrupts the career of a private citizen, that is unpleasant for him and his family. But what about the men who hold high public office, whose words and deeds affect the fate of nations? What happens when their memories fail, their tempers flare, and their health declines, when they become incapable of properly using the power they hold?

Napoleon Bonaparte was born in 1769, and at the age of twenty-six married his first wife, Josephine, who was then thirty-two. To all appearances they lived happily together during his rise to power. He became emperor in 1804, and he and Josephine went through a new religious ceremony to confirm their marriage. Then in October 1809 he ordered the door between their apartments walled up and in December 1809 had their marriage annulled, ostensibly so that he could make a political marriage, one that would strengthen France's position in Europe.

We may question whether that was his real motive. Since 1807 or thereabouts he had been conducting love affairs with girls young enough to be his daughters. In November 1809 (before the annulment) he had proposed to Anna, sister of the Tsar of Russia, a girl of only fifteen years to his forty. He was rejected. In February 1810 he proposed to eighteen-year-old Marie Louise, daughter of the Emperor of Austria, and was accepted.

Now there occurred an extraordinary encounter between the

Empress and one of Napoleon's girl friends. Early in 1807 at a ball in Warsaw, Napoleon (then still married to Josephine) had met Maria Walewska, the seventeen-year-old wife of an elderly Polish nobleman. He fell madly in love with her and promptly blabbed of his infatuation to many of his own staff and to the whole of the Polish provisional government. (How like Charles Dickens's public confession.) At his second private meeting with Maria, Napoleon frightened her so badly that she fainted; he raped her while she lay unconscious.

Despite this unromantic beginning, Maria grew to love Napoleon; over the next few years she spent much time with him, and on May 4, 1810, she bore him a son, Alexandre. Napoleon promptly presented Maria and her baby to his new Empress Marie Louise! (Again, how like Dickens's introduction of his mistress to his wife.)

Up until 1807 Napoleon had enjoyed exceptionally good physical health; he endured without any apparent ill effects the hardships of his military campaigns. He was also exceptionally quick-thinking and decisive—an important factor in his successes as general in war and administrator in peace. But not long after he began chasing young girls, he began to manifest uncharacteristic signs of physical weakness and lapses of mental ability. Of course, we do not know about all his spells of sickness; yet some of them, because they occurred on important occasions when Napoleon was in the public eye, have been reported in detail.

On September 5, 1812, two days before the battle of Borodino, Napoleon felt ill. His legs were swollen and he had difficulty urinating. On September 6 he had what has been described as a "feverish chill," presumably alternate spells of feeling hot and cold. Walking about to look over the Russian battle lines, he was seen to lean against the wheel of a gun and press his head on the rim. Some onlookers thought he was trying to cool his forehead on the iron tire; it is just as likely that he was clinging to the gun because he had temporarily lost his sense of balance. The symptoms continued on September 7, the day of the battle; his pulse was high and irregular. On September 8 he had difficulty in controlling his hands to such a degree that he could not write.

In October 1813, before the battle of Leipzig, he showed extreme torpor and inactivity. On October 10 he did no work at all. During the battle he had a high temperature and showed complete indifference to what was going on. From the evening of October 16 to the night of October 18, he did not give a single order.

In 1815, after his return from Elba, he showed uncharacteristic spells of drowsiness: Sometimes he would fall asleep over a book, and sometimes he would sleep fifteen hours at a stretch. Even during the battle of Waterloo (June 18, 1815), when one would have expected Napoleon to be at his most alert and energetic, he suffered drowsy spells!

In July 1815 he was seen to be experiencing spells of sweating. At St. Helena he suffered shivering fits: At times, even in warm weather, he had fires lit and took hot baths, trying to keep warm.

After this time, and with the scanty medical records that are available, one cannot dogmatize about Napoleon's health. Yet the incidents mentioned above do suggest that, from his late thirties on, he suffered rather severely from emotional and physical symptoms typical of the male climacteric. If he had not experienced those symptoms, the future of Europe would have been radically different.

Thus far I have described how the climacteric affects a man's sex life and his work. But men have other functions and relationships: They are voters and taxpayers and members of clubs and religions; they must deal with friends, store clerks, policemen, and landlords; they are constantly being influenced by, and constantly reacting upon, the society in which they live.

By the time they reach their forties, most men have made a passable adjustment to society; they may not always be happy and contented; yet they have found how to make a living, are getting some pleasure from life, and are not robbing banks or blowing up police stations. But in many cases the climacteric can sharply derange the man-society relationship, sometimes with serious results for both.

Men who lose libido or potency at the climacteric usually try to keep it secret because if it became known, they fear that they would suffer a severe loss of face among their male and female acquaintances. This is so because fertility in men and women has in most societies and at most times been honored; sterility and impotence have been scorned, even punished. "He that is wounded in the stones, or hath his privy member cut off, shall not enter into the congregation of the Lord," says the Bible (Deuteronomy 23:1). The man whose testicles were injured or whose penis was cut off was barred from religious worship.

POTENCY FOR SALE

In Chapter 1 I described the various forms of impotence. These symptoms have been common for thousands of years, and for thousands of years uncounted millions of men have desperately sought relief. The demand for treatment created the supply, so farmers, fishermen, hunters, pharmacists, physicians, priests, and magicians, to name but a few, began and have continued to produce and sell aphrodisiac foods, beverages, drugs, and charms.

In ancient times middle-aged Syrians bathed in young men's blood and Romans drank gladiators' blood in the hope of regaining their lost manhood. Ovid (43 B.C.–A.D. 17) described the use of aphrodisiacs in his *Remedia Amoris*. Pope Innocent VIII (1484–92) died after receiving transfusions of blood from three young men. Paracelsus (1493–1541), a Swiss alchemist and physician, concocted an "elixir of life" that was supposed to rejuvenate old men.

The horn of the Indian rhinoceros looks something like an erect penis; when ground into powder, this horn long has been in great demand as an aphrodisiac, and in some parts of the world it still is. An onion or garlic bulb, with its stiff stalk, looks something like a human scrotum surmounted by an erect penis; so these vegetables were, and in some places are still, eaten to restore lost virility. So is the thick, stiff root of the ginseng plant, which is still being grown in the United States for export to the Orient. Mandrake roots often assume grotesque, man-like shapes, so men eat them to become more manly. The tomato, when first introduced to Europe, was called the "love apple" because of its supposed aphrodisiac properties.

Cantharides (kan-thar'-i-deez) or "Spanish fly" (actually the pulverized bodies of *Cantharis vesicatoria* beetles) is a famous old aphrodisiac. Alexander Pope (1688–1744) in his poem *January and May* tells of the sixty-year-old knight who took a young wife; on his wedding night the prudent bridegroom doses himself with several aphrodisiacs, including sea holly and cantharides. Spanish fly is a powerful irritant to the genitourinary system and can indeed produce an erection of the penis. The problem in using it is to draw the line between an effective and a lethal dose. One man's treat may be another man's poison.

Yohimbine (yo-him'-been), prepared from the bark of the *Corynanthe* (kor-in-anth'-ee) *yohimbe* tree, has been successfully used on bulls and stallions but is dangerous for men. The oyster has enjoyed a long-standing, though unjustified, reputation as an aphrodisiac. In France Dr. Charles Brown Ségard (1814–94) tried injecting himself with an extract of dogs' testicles.

In the nineteenth century, the development of mass-production techniques, steam transportation, and newspaper and billboard advertising encouraged the vending of many allegedly aphrodisiac medicines. Aromatic Lozenges of Steel, Turkish Wafers, and Mormon Elders' Damiana Wafers offered American males an enjoyable, invigorating conquest of their sexual weaknesses.

Helmbold's Extract of Buchu was advertised in the 1860s as a cure for a long list of ailments, including "Disorganization or Paralysis of the Organs of Generation." Walker's California Vinegar Bitters used the slogan "Vinegar Bitters Is All the Go for

Love!" Pendleton's Calisaya Tonic Bitters were advertised as a cure for "Impaired or Exhausted Vital Energy."

Most of the liquid aphrodisiacs—even the "temperance bitters" marketed for teetotalers—contained high proportions of alcohol, some as high as 40 percent or more. Such medicine had the usual effect that Shakespeare ascribed to ordinary alcoholic drink: "It provokes the desire, but takes away the performance." Some manufacturers offered ointments for the patient to rub into his testicles and penis. Some of these were just colored, perfumed cold cream or petroleum jelly; others contained powerful irritants, such as red pepper!

Sir John Hampton's Vital Restorative used a clever bit of applied psychology. These pills contained the dye methylene blue, which turned the patient's urine green. This made him think that his genitourinary system was undergoing a thorough, beneficial cleansing. Organo Tablets were advertised as containing an extract of ram's testicles. (There is still, by the way, a brisk market in the Orient for dried seals' testicles, collected at the annual seal harvest on the Pribiloff Islands.) "Magnetic belts" were sold; they contained a number of small magnets which, being worn day and night close to one's body, were supposed to restore "vital power."

Individual physicians have continued to experiment. Dr. Elie Metchnikov (1845–1916), deputy director of the Pasteur Institute, prescribed doses of yogurt; in the 1920s Dr. S. Vornonov was implanting monkeys' testicles in men who sought rejuvenation. Dr. Wilhelm Reich, a pupil of Freud, was in the 1950s putting patients inside a metal-lined box, the Orgone Accumulator, that supposedly focused cosmic energy to heighten their orgasmic abilities.

Today the impotent man can buy gadgets that give electric shocks to his penis, vibrators that will massage it, and lamps that bathe it in ultraviolet or infrared radiation. An overdose of the ultraviolet light might leave the user with a sunburned penis; otherwise such gadgets are not likely to do much harm.

As for pills and potions, the present-day aphrodisiac is likely to be a vitamin-mineral mixture designed to cure the patient's supposed state of malnutrition. It will probably be expensive. At the time of writing, a "Super Strength Sex Aid" tablet, containing fourteen vitamins and ten minerals "Plus the Amazing RED VITAMIN" (whatever that is), is being sold by mail at 60 for $5; comparable vitamin-mineral tablets in the drugstore are priced at 240 for $5. Sometimes a patent medicine, ostensibly marketed for some other complaint, gets a word-of-mouth reputation as an aphrodisiac: this happened with Hadacol in the 1950s.

But despite all the claims and rumors, there is no safe, legal drug or apparatus that will produce any direct effect on the erection mechanism of the penis. (There *is* one nonchemical, non-mechanical aphrodisiac that is both safe and effective, which I shall describe later in the book.) Nevertheless, the sale and purchase of aphrodisiacs will probably never cease because, even if the pill or gadget is in itself useless, the user's faith in it may quite likely produce the desired results. The reason for this is that about 98 percent of impotence cases are of psychological origin. Not all of these men can conjure up the requisite intensity of faith; yet some tests with placebos* have yielded improvement in 35 percent of impotent patients.

HEALTH FOR SALE

Quite apart from the special problem of impotence, middle-aged men have good reason to take thought for their general health. In the United States the death rate of males from fifty to sixty-nine years of age is 50 percent higher than that for females.

Suppose a man—perhaps after decades of generally good health —experiences an assortment of the distressing symptoms of the climacteric; he is tempted to self-diagnosis and self-medication. He is perhaps influenced by the flood of books, magazine articles, and advertisements that offer quick, certain cures for whatever ails

---

* Placebo (pla-see'-bo) is a substance that the patient believes will benefit him but that in fact is inert and has of itself no therapeutic action.

him. He decides that this kind of pill or that special diet is just what's needed to make him feel like his old self again. (Raymond Hull, in the Introduction, tells how he dosed himself with vitamins. Perhaps they did him no harm; yet he might have had better results if he had sought medical advice sooner.)

Some of the medicines and foodstuffs offered for sale are simply placebos; some of them, harmless in small doses, may be dangerous if taken in large quantities; some of the fad diets may be injurious if followed for a long time. In many cases the principal risk of such remedies is that the man's faith in them, his stubborn hope that they will eventually produce a cure, may lead to a dangerous delay in obtaining qualified advice and treatment.

ANTISOCIAL BEHAVIOR

Loss of virility is by no means the only unwelcome effect of the climacteric. There may be changes for the worse in the man's relationship with friends and fellow workers and with the whole society he lives in.

A man describes a "lack of confidence in my own abilities and others, sense of futility with life, a strong cynicism combined with an extreme restlessness." The spells of bad temper that are a common symptom of the climacteric will obviously cause problems for the man at work and with his friends. In extreme cases they may lead to quarrels, fights, even murders.

In the Bible the first book of Samuel tells the story of Saul, King of Israel. In his middle age Saul began to be afflicted from time to time by "an evil spirit." At first the evil spirit merely produced spells of depression, which could be relieved by Saul's listening to music.

A little later, Saul began to have fits of homicidal rage; he repeatedly tried to kill David, the handsome young harpist and military hero. One of these attempted murders is described in chapter 18, verse 11: David was playing the harp before Saul who, as seems to have been his custom, had a javelin in his hand. "And

Saul cast the javelin; for he said, I will smite David even to the wall with it. And David avoided out of his presence twice."

Between homicidal spells Saul would be reconciled with David. "As the Lord liveth, he shall not be slain" (I Sam. 9:6). Then a little later, in person or by emissaries, he would be after David's blood again. Saul next turned against his own son Jonathan, accused him of a homosexual relationship with David, and tried to kill him, too, with the ever-handy javelin (I Sam. 20:30–33).

PHYSICAL SYMPTOMS

Spells of dizziness and light-headedness may lead to accident, injury, and death if they occur at inopportune times—for example, when one is driving a car. Some physical symptoms, such as essential hypertension and heart irregularities, may be detected during medical examinations and may cause difficulties for the man who is seeking life insurance or whose job requires a high level of physical fitness.

MENTAL AND EMOTIONAL SYMPTOMS

Consider the results on a man's social life when he begins to have frequent lapses of memory. New acquaintances, whether business or social, feel slighted when he cannot remember their names; how much more put out old friends may be when he forgets theirs. Weakened memory impairs the man's ability at, and enjoyment of, games such as chess and bridge, in which success depends to a large extent on memory.

For a man who has to do mental work, memory lapses are a serious handicap. If he has to keep turning to reference books for information that he should already know and remember, if he is always writing notes to himself as reminders of what he has to do, if he continually forgets his bright ideas before he can act upon them, he is obviously at a disadvantage compared with men whose memories are unimpaired.

In addition, there are the potentially grave effects of memory lapses if a man has to appear as witness or defendant in a court of law or is called to give testimony before a legislative committee. When the man in this position says, "I can't remember," it may be assumed that he is lying.

Consider the example that Raymond Hull mentioned in the Introduction, in which he had completely forgotten the identity of the woman he was working with. Suppose, that day, on the witness stand, he had been asked, "What do you know about Olga Ruskin?" He would have had to reply, "I know nothing about her. I've never heard of her." "But here's a letter that you wrote to her this morning." "I don't remember writing any such letter. I can't say what's in it, or who the woman is to whom it's addressed." The letter is read, Hull's signature is shown, and he is branded a clumsy perjurer; yet, to the best of his recollection at the time, he would have been telling the truth.

THE CLIMACTERIC IN PUBLIC LIFE

In most countries nearly all high political and administrative offices are filled by men. Women's susceptibility to the emotional and intellectual upheavals of the menopause has often been cited as a reason for excluding them from such high positions. But what about the men?

Consider the career of Benito Mussolini. A comparison of the earlier and latter parts of his life suggests that he may have experienced the male climacteric in a severe form.

Before he came to eminence as a politician, he was a brilliant newspaperman: Between the ages of twenty-nine and thirty-two he more than tripled the circulation of Milan's daily *Avanti* and then founded *Il Popolo d'Italia*, soon increasing its circulation to 100,000.

In October 1922 he worked to avoid bloodshed during and after the fascist March on Rome. In a few months, after the fascist coup, he reorganized the civil service, made the trains run on time, and greatly reduced public expenditure. In his personal life he was very thrifty: Although he held several ministerial posts, he did not even draw the full salary for one. In 1923 he began negotiations to resolve the bitter, fifty-three-year-old dispute between the Catholic Church and the Kingdom of Italy and in 1929 signed the Lateran Treaty and Concordat.

By the end of his first ten years in power he had built hundreds of bridges and thousands of kilometers of roads; he had drained marshes, irrigated regions of scanty rainfall, increased agricultural production, expanded Italy's merchant marine, reorganized the social insurance system, and broken the power of the Mafia. It could fairly be said that, during this period, he was a prodigy of efficiency and decisiveness.

During this time, too, Mussolini enjoyed vigorous health and was very virile. A devoted family man with three sons and two daughters, he also had many hasty, casual sexual encounters with women. Then, in his late forties, he began to show signs of physical, emotional, and mental deterioration.

By the age of forty-seven, he was suffering from chronic dyspepsia; he ate a frugal diet, and drank neither wine nor coffee, yet was racked with pain after every meal. He later developed a severe stomach ulcer.

At forty-nine he fell in love with Claretta Pettacci, a doctor's daughter twenty-nine years younger than himself. After four years' pining for her, he took the extraordinary step of interviewing her mother and formally asking Signora Pettacci's permission to make Claretta his mistress.

Mussolini had for some time been showing a nearly grotesque degree of personal vanity. He refused to celebrate, or even to let the press mention, his fiftieth birthday; to conceal his increasing baldness, he took to shaving his head.

His political judgment began to falter. For years Mussolini had condemned anti-Semitism as a typical piece of Hitler's stupidity ("He's quite mad," said Mussolini), and Italy gave asylum to many German-Jewish refugees. Suddenly, at age fifty-five, he reversed this policy, issued his Aryan Manifesto, and started persecuting Jews.

He began to concern himself with trifles—for example, banning tea drinking for party members or auditioning drum majors. He became hopelessly indecisive, vacillating on major policy issues (he reversed himself several times on relations with Germany and Britain).

There is no need to describe in detail his weak, ineffective management of Italy's war effort; but one astounding personal incident is worth mentioning. For twelve years Mussolini had concealed from his wife Rachele his liaison with Claretta. In 1944 Rachele found out about it, and Mussolini actually permitted an interview between his wife and his mistress. (There is a startling similarity here with the conduct of Napoleon and Charles Dickens.)

One cannot, of course, obtain full medical details about such famous figures as Mussolini. Yet what has been made public does suggest that he may have experienced the male climacteric in a fairly severe form.

Not only dictators are subject to the climacteric. In the democratic system as we know it, a high proportion of candidates for public office are men of ages prone to the climacteric. I must emphasize, once again, that not all men experience the climacteric. Yet many of them do. I would not propose that men of this age group be barred from public office; yet it might be worthwhile to suggest that such men are not necessarily the best or the only people to be considered for office.

What may be the results if the abilities have been lessened and the personalities changed in many of our middle-aged public men by the effects of the male climacteric? I shall suggest in Chapter 8 some precautions that might be taken to guard against such risks.

Part II
CAUSES OF
THE CLIMACTERIC

In Part II, I shall describe some possible causes of the climacteric. Chapters 4, 5, and 6 deal, respectively, with physical, psychological, and social causes. I would not suggest, however, that these categories can be strictly separated for study or for treatment. For example, suppose that for some physical reason—say alcoholic intoxication—a man discovers that he has become impotent. That first failure may become the psychological cause for additional failures after the man has sobered up. Thus, there will in practice be some interaction between these categories.

Not all these causes will be operative in any one man. I mention that fact because I don't want the next three chapters to have a needlessly depressing effect on readers. However, we rarely see a case in which only *one* cause is operative. So it is important to identify all the causes in each case so that adequate treatment and, where necessary, self-treatment can be recommended.

4
Physical Causes

In Chapter I I pointed out some of the ways in which the symptoms of the male climacteric differ from those of female menopause. The two syndromes differ not only in their natures but also in their causes.

Some medical writers deny that there is any physical cause for the male climacteric: They say that because some men do not exprience the climacteric at all and because those who do experience it show such a wide variety of symptoms, the causes must all be emotional.

Yet consider the menopause. Some women simply stop menstruating and show no other symptoms at all; some women have a few, mild symptoms; some exhibit certain symptoms that are undoubtedly of emotional origin along with others that have a physical cause. One might as well cite these variations to prove that the menopausal women are not undergoing any physical change.

WHAT'S NOT THE CAUSE

A former hospital orderly writes: "I have come across a few men who claimed they had no further sexual desires after middle age. . . . Some claimed that their overindulgence in the sex act, particularly after marriage stretching over ten to twenty years, was to blame for their revulsion or indifference later." I would emphasize that male sexuality is not like a pair of shoes that wears out with use: it could more aptly be compared with the ability to play chess—the more you do it, the better you become. Sexual abstinence, indeed, leads to more problems than does so-called over-indulgence.

For the grown man, sexual desire and sexual response are not so much a hormonal as an emotional function. Maintenance of sexuality does not depend upon conserving a limited quantity of hormones or of sperm; it depends upon creating and maintaining a favorable psychoneurological condition.

Many men who fear that they have worn out their sexuality and lapsed permanently into impotence can be reassured by the fact that they often experience morning erections. Until recently, the morning erection was not considered as evidence of the man's sexuality; it was thought to be caused simply by the pressure of urine in a full bladder (although, as far as I know, nobody commented on the fact that for these men a full bladder during the day did not produce an erection).

However, recent research on sleep has shown that most men actually obtain several erections each night in the rapid-eye-movement (REM) periods during which dreams are experienced. If the man happens to wake up during, or immediately after, a REM period, he still has the erection that was produced by the emotional activity of that period.

For the impotent man, this provides proof that he has not worn out his ability to produce and sustain an erection: He can do it in REM sleep, so he can, with suitable treatment, regain the ability to do it when he is awake.

Hormone and sperm production may, in some men, decline at midlife. But I would repeat that this does not indicate the near-exhaustion of a limited stock; it is merely caused by the slowing down of production processes that can, in most cases, easily be restored to full vigor.

HORMONES

A hormone (derived from the Greek word *hormaien*, which means to arouse or to stimulate) may be thought of as a chemical messenger that is produced by one of the ductless (endocrine) glands and is carried by the blood to other parts of the body, which it stimulates to action. First, I will briefly describe the most important hormone-secreting glands in the human body and their functions.

The pituitary gland is near the base of the brain and is an integral part of it. The pituitary has many functions; the one that relates to male sexuality is described later in this chapter.

The thyroid gland is in the neck, just below the larynx. Improper functioning of the thyroid in infants may produce dwarfism or cretinism. Thyroid deficiency in adults produces myxedema (mik-se-dee'-ma)—low body temperature, dry skin, and sluggish mental processes. Overactivity of the thyroid produces Graves's disease—rapid heartbeat, nervousness, and weight loss. An enlarged thyroid (caused by lack of iodine in the diet) produces the swollen neck of goiter.

The thymus gland, in the upper chest, controls several aspects of development in infancy and adolescence; it disintegrates at adulthood. (In animals, this gland is called the sweetbread.)

The pancreas, near the stomach, has a dual function. One part of it discharges pancreatic juice into the intestine, where it aids digestion. The endocrine part of the pancreas produces the hormone insulin, which controls the use of sugar in the body. Failure of this function causes the well-known disease diabetes mellitus (sugar diabetes).

The two adrenals (or suprarenal glands) lie on top of the kidneys. They produce the hormones adrenalin and cortisone, which control the body's defensive reactions to stress.

The sex glands (gonads) are the ovaries in women and the testicles in men. Their best-known functions are to produce the ova (eggs) and the sperm (seed) by which the human species reproduces itself. But they also produce hormones, the most important of which are estrogen in women and testosterone in men.

In normal conditions all these glands work together to maintain a balance in the internal environment of our bodies—the balance that gives us the physical and emotional experience of "good health." Poetically inclined biologists sometimes compare this system with an orchestra, in which all the musicians combine to produce the harmony of life. Now let us see how, in some cases, that harmony may be turned into discord.

THE SEX HORMONE SYSTEM

One major cause for the changes experienced by the woman at menopause is a rapid, severe decline in the level of the female hormones (estrogens). This decline produces a correspondingly rapid sexual involution—a reversal of the sexual development she experienced at puberty. Her physical femininity, so to speak, is reduced: She can never again bear a child; in the eyes of some men, perhaps, she may be less sexually attractive. For others who do not want the worry and expense of fatherhood, a woman unable to bear a child might be *more* attractive. (There is not necessarily any decline in a woman's sex drive due to menopause: Indeed, it may well increase because she no longer has any fear of pregnancy.) In contrast, the great majority of men experience no such severe hormonal change in midlife. Let us look at this system that regulates man's sexuality, briefly examine its normal operation, and see what, in some cases, may derange its functioning.

We are primarily concerned here with two hormones that are sometimes referred to as gonadotrophins (gō-nad-e-trō'-fin) (meaning that they travel to, and act upon, the gonads, or sex glands). They are produced by the pituitary gland, which is located immediately below the brain. The pituitary has two lobes, the anterior (foremost) and posterior (hindmost); the anterior lobe produces these two hormones. Exactly the same two hormones are produced in men and women, and in both sexes they serve corresponding functions. The principal difference is that in men these hormones are produced as often as necessary whereas in women, between puberty and menopause, the two hormones are released about once a month and are responsible for the menstrual cycle.

LH (Luteinizing Hormone)

In women LH acts upon the corpus luteum, the part of the ovary that produces the female hormone progesterone, which has to do with childbearing. In men LH acts upon the part of the testicle, the interstitial cells, that produces the most important of the male hormones, testosterone. Some writers, when referring to men, use the term ICSH (interstitial cell stimulating hormone), instead of LH, although chemically there is no difference.

FSH (Follicle Stimulating Hormone)

In women FSH stimulates the ovaries to produce eggs. (The "follicles" are the egg-generating cells.) In men FSH stimulates the parts of the testicles that produce sperm (the seminiferous tubules).

Testosterone

Testosterone is the most important of several hormones called the androgens (from the Greek *andros*, meaning man, and *gennaien*, meaning to create). Already, in the mother's womb, the androgens determine that the developing embryo is going to be a boy. (In the absence of androgens, the embryo becomes a girl.)

During puberty testosterone causes development of male sex characteristics—the masculine build, the deep voice, the growth of beard and body hair, and so on. Administration of male hormones to females can noticeably increase their sex drive. For example, a woman who is receiving testosterone (with or without an admixture of estrogen) for the treatment of breast cancer or certain

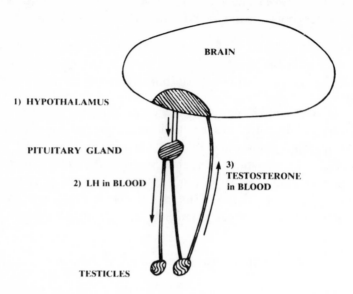

Production and action of Luteinizing Hormone LH
(1) Hypothalamus monitors testosterone level in blood and "orders" pituitary to produce hormone LH. (2) LH is carried via bloodstream to testicles, to give the order to produce testosterone. (3) Testosterone is carried via bloodstream back to hypothalamus, showing that the original order has been obeyed.

types of menopausal problems, may abandon her traditional feminine sex role and start aggressively initiating sexual activities. I have heard of cases in which the husband comes to his wife's physician and complains, "Doctor, you've *got* to stop this medicine you're giving my wife. I just can't take it any longer!"

Experiments with animals suggest that male sex hormones determine certain forms of behavior that are commonly thought to be unrelated to sex. Among barnyard fowl, for example, there is a rigid "pecking order": The hen at the top pecks all the others and is pecked by none; the hen at the bottom is pecked by all the others and may not peck any of them in return. But give that bottom hen an injection of testosterone, and as the hormone takes effect, she rebels and becomes number one.

There is much the same phenomenon with cows: They have an invariable "marching order," with the boss cow at the head and the humblest cow at the tail of the line. But give that last cow a testosterone treatment, and she will very soon take over the lead!

Is it the same with men? Could a decline of testosterone production diminish a man's self-confidence? Could that be detected, consciously or unconsciously, by other people, so that his status is lowered in the family, on the job, or in his political party? Could that hormone decline have other emotional effects, as yet unsuspected, on his personal feelings or on his relations with other people? At present, we don't know. But I ask the questions to suggest that the midlife change may be considerably more complex than just a reduction of the man's sex drive.

The Hypothalamus

I said that the hormones LH and FSH, among others, are produced and passed into the bloodstream by the pituitary gland. But the anterior pituitary does not work independently: It is controlled by the hypothalamus, an area in the lower front part of the brain. The connection between the two is by a stalk that carries a rich blood supply.

The hypothalamus might be compared with a factory computer that constantly takes readings from various points in the production line; it keeps tab on the stock of raw materials and finished products in hand; it takes note of orders coming in from the sales staff; and from time to time it receives fresh directives from the manager's office. On the basis of all this information, it controls the entire production process to achieve optimum results.

In the male body, if not enough testosterone is being made, the hypothalamus orders the pituitary to produce LH; the LH goes to the testicles and stimulates the interstitial cells to produce more testosterone. Once a sufficient level of testosterone has been attained in the blood, the hypothalamus detects it and orders the pituitary to stop producing LH. The interstitial cells then cease production until the testosterone level in the blood falls low enough to alert the hypothalamus, starting the cycle again.

The hypothalamus also responds to emotional changes. If a man is feeling anxious or depressed, for example, his hypothalamus may order his pituitary to reduce, or temporarily stop, sending out the hormones LH and FSH; then his testicles halt production of testosterone. That is one of the reasons why, at times of emotional stress, a man may temporarily lose his sex drive.

So the hypothalamus acts as a link between the nervous system and the endocrine system. It controls many basic drives such as hunger, thirst, and libido; it regulates blood pressure, heart rate, body temperature, and water balance in the human body.

HORMONE DECLINE

Men in their late forties or fifties begin to show signs of slightly diminishing androgen levels; but usually there is no such definite or profound change as the rapid estrogen decrease in menopausal women. For 85 percent of men the hormonal change is hardly noticeable. Their libido and fertility may be somewhat reduced but are certainly not terminated. (Charles Chaplin fathered a child at 72; Goethe at 82.) For this large majority of men, sexual involution, or loss of masculinity, is quite gradual—so slow, indeed, that many of them are scarcely aware of any change.

But about 15 percent of men do experience a sudden decline of androgen output, caused by rapid, premature aging of the testicles. These men suffer a sharp diminution, or complete loss, of libido, a marked change of temperament (for example, unaccustomed passivity and lack of drive), and a higher-than-average incidence of psychosomatic symptoms.

Low production of testosterone and sperm in an aging testicle will lead to high levels of gonadotrophins—LH and FSH—in the man's bloodstream. The pituitary keeps pouring out these two hormones to stimulate production, but its messages are ignored, or only feebly answered, by the testicles.

I emphasize, though, that this rapid, sharp decline of testosterone and sperm production is *not* a normal part of the aging process; it occurs in only 15 percent of middle-aged men. (It may also occasionally be found in much younger men.) For most men, then, the midlife crisis probably has little or nothing to do with sex hormones.

GENERAL PHYSICAL DETERIORATION

By the time they reach the half-century mark, many men are beginning to feel and to show signs of bodily wear and tear (medically referred to as degenerative changes). One experiences a general decrease of physical strength and vigor, a diminishing elasticity and flexibility, because all the cells in his body are aging to a greater or lesser extent.

This process of aging of tissues and cells is almost a reversal of the process of adolescence. During the formative years, the specific functions of the various tissues develop to maximum efficiency (evolution); during middle and old age, cell efficiency and tissue quality gradually decrease (involution). Quite likely, a lot of things begin to go wrong at once. The following are the most common of these nonhormonal, nonsex-linked physical changes.

Deterioration of Muscles

Muscle fibers are elastic, contractile cells that shorten and thicken when activated and lengthen again when deactivated. (A well-known example is the shortening and thickening of the biceps when the arm is bent.) Even when not consciously activated, muscles maintain a certain "tone" or firmness that is at a maximum in youth and lessens with age. Muscle tone is important, for example, in keeping one's balance and maintaining an erect posture; as muscle tone decreases, the man begins to slump or stoop. Another typical middle-age phenomenon is the potbelly; the man's diaphragm and abdominal muscles are slackening, so his abdomen begins to protrude.

Exercise tolerance lessens with age: The muscles respond more slowly when demands are made upon them and tire more quickly. The muscles, if not regularly used, may even atrophy—diminish in substance or number of cells.

One cannot predict the exact age at which muscular deterioration will set in for any individual, but observation of men engaged in arduous jobs and sports (boxing, bull fighting, and football) shows that the change is generally noticeable by the mid-thirties.

The muscles that produce ejaculation are not exempt from this general weakening; as a man gets into midlife, he may find that his semen oozes out instead of spurting in a powerful jet, as it did when he was in his sexual prime. (The reduced pressure, though, does not impair the man's chances of fathering a child.)

Deterioration of Arteries

Efficient blood circulation depends not only on the pumping power of the heart but also on the active elasticity of the arterial walls, which expand or contract in response to greater or lesser blood demand.

The middle-aged man, as a rule, shows a noticeable hardening of his arteries (arteriosclerosis) caused by loss of elasticity of the arterial walls and deposits of cholesterol and fats in the arterial walls. These deposits begin at an earlier age in men than in women, and by middle age can reach harmful proportions. (Women seem to be protected by estrogens from early hardening of the arteries, but many of them succumb to it later on.)

Sclerotic (from the Greek *skleros*, meaning dry or hard) arteries cannot adjust to pressure changes because they are somewhat like rusty pipes. The man's blood pressure may rise, he finds that he cannot tolerate vigorous exercise (when muscles are demanding an increased blood supply); poor circulation in his heart muscle may cause angina pectoris, a severe pain in the midchest that radiates to the neck or left arm and is brought on by physical exertion.

Among the most striking changes that the twentieth century has seen in the disease pattern of Western societies has been the emergence of coronary artery disease as one of the most common killers of middle-aged men. The reason for this increase is not altogether clear. Several factors may be involved, including high intake of animal fats and sugar, lack of exercise, and excessive tobacco smoking.

Deterioration of Lung Tissue

The healthy young human lung somewhat resembles a football bladder encased in a basket. The diaphragm and the respiratory muscles between the ribs and around the rib cage alternately expand and compress the lungs, taking in and expelling air, to oxygenate and ventilate the blood.

But in many middle-aged men, the elasticity of this system is much reduced. The lung capacity ("vital capacity" is the medical textbook term) decreases. His intake of oxygen and output of carbon dioxide are slower and smaller in volume.

Most of the time—sitting at a desk or riding in an automobile— the man probably notices no sign of this lung deterioration. But if he has some extra exertion—walking up four flights of stairs, shoveling snow off the driveway—he gets badly out of breath. Also unknown to him, his shallow, inefficient breathing results in poor oxygenation of all his tissues and so speeds the general process of degeneration.

Degeneration of Joints and Ligaments

Because of their construction and constant use, the joints are very vulnerable to wear and tear. They are composed of cartilage-lined bone junctions, held together by ligaments, capsules, and muscle tendons (sinews). The spinal column has twenty-four inter-vertebral joints in which the intervertebral cartilages or disks function as sockets and shock absorbers at the same time.

Degeneration of joint structures does not necessarily indicate any disease or injury: In many men it is a result of the ordinary wear and tear of life—the never-ending struggle against gravity, the millions of little jolts caused by walking, automobile riding, playing games, and so on.

The cartilage joint linings and the intervertebral disks wear thin or, in some spots, break down completely. The ligaments, capsules, and tendons lose some of their elasticity and become slack, rigid, or calcified. Then joint movement becomes painful; the back is held more stiffly. The middle-aged man gradually loses the flexibility of youth and assumes the stiffness of old age.

Aging Nervous System

The nervous system—the brain, spinal cord, peripheral nerves, and autonomic nervous system—begins to show signs of wear and tear by middle age. The nervous system is composed of the actual nerve cells (neurons) and the nerve fibers or tracts (dendrites). (In the brain the former are called "gray matter," the latter "white matter.")

Some nerve cells actively generate electrical impulses that travel along the fibers to the body's target organs for action (for example, telling the erection mechanism of the penis to begin). Other cells receive nerve stimuli or messages from the organs or body periphery and respond to them appropriately, according to the body's needs (for example, a sensation of heat from the skin activates the temperature-control mechanism). The nerve cells could be likened to electrical generators and receptors and the nerve fibers to a network of wires conveying electrical impulses.

The central nervous system has a voluntary and an involuntary (autonomic) part. The autonomic nervous system is itself divided into two sections, serving different functions: the sympathetic or activating system and the parasympathetic or restorative system.

Like other parts of the body, the sex organs are supplied by both the sympathetic and parasympathetic nervous systems. The sympathetic system is concerned with ejaculation; it sends branches to the right and left pelvic plexuses. The parasympathetic system controls erection of the penis.

At the pelvic plexuses the sympathetic and parasympathetic nerve fibers join to form the so-called nervi erigentes (nur'-vee eri-jent'-ees); division or destruction of these fibers can lead to permanent impotence. Any proposal for surgery that might injure these structures should be carefully studied and discussed between doctor and patient. There are three operations that can cause impotence: radical perineal prostatectomy (this is only one of several possible types of surgery to the prostate gland); abdominoperineal resection for cancer of the rectum; and sympathectomy (cutting the main nerve trunk alongside the spinal cord as treatment for certain problems with leg circulation). Men should know, however, that a secondary impotence of this nature does *not* necessarily produce total sexual inability. Prospects for a continued, satisfactory sex life for such men are discussed in Chapter 7.

Surgery of the kind mentioned above is by no means common. Yet all men will experience with time a gradual deterioration of the nervous system. In a radio receiver or transmitter, the materials and wires wear with prolonged use, so it is with the human nervous system; the creation of energy and the transmission of impulses eventually become more sluggish and less efficient.

Most parts of the body have the ability to renew themselves by cell division: One old cell splits to form two new ones. Nerve cells cannot reproduce themselves this way; when one of them is worn out, it simply dies. Thus, the number of living, active cells in the nervous system, including the brain, is gradually decreasing.

Typical effects of this deterioration are loss of speed and skill in reflex and voluntary movements. For example, one may become less nimble in regaining his balance after a stumble (a reflex movement), or one may notice that his piano playing or handball playing are becoming slower and less accurate (essentially voluntary movements).

Signs of aging of the brain may be seen as early in life as fifty. The metabolism (inner combustion) of the brain cells begins to decline; as a result, the blood flow to the brain is reduced. Usually one cannot point to any one part of the brain as the site of damage; there is just a general decline of cerebral efficiency. This decline is a probable cause for several of the symptoms described in Chapter I: dizzy spells, irritability, fatigue, moodiness or depression, weakened mental ability (memory, concentration, decisiveness, and so on), and loss of self-confidence.

Enlargement of Prostate Gland

The normal function of the prostate gland is to produce seminal fluid, in which the sperm are carried forward to the penis for ejaculation. (This somewhat resembles the transportation by pipeline of mineral particles mixed into a slurry with water.)

In some middle-aged men hormonal changes cause a thickening of certain parts of the prostate. The enlarged prostate, because of its position surrounding the urethra (the outlet of the bladder), begins to obstruct the flow of urine, causing the irregularities mentioned in Chapter I. The aging prostate also reduces to some extent its production of seminal fluid, so the man's ejaculations lessen in volume. (At the same time, the ejaculatory muscles of the pelvic floor and spermatic cord get weaker, so the pressure of ejaculations, too, is reduced.)

Eye Changes

For most people eyesight begins to gradually deteriorate quite early in life. At first the changes are slight and unnoticed; but by midlife defects may be apparent.

One common change is a progressive slackening of adaptor muscles, producing farsightedness: The eye's focal point is farther away; one can see well at a distance but for nearby objects, as in reading, writing, or close-up work, must strain the eyes to focus or perhaps cannot focus the eyes at all without spectacles.

Moreover, the lens of the eye tends to lose some of its elasticity: The muscles that modify its curvature become weaker and sluggish. So, the middle-aged eye adjusts more slowly than it used to. The man now experiences difficulty in any activity that requires rapid eye adjustment. Jobs requiring quick changes from near to distant vision become difficult or impossible; in games that require rapid eye adaptation, such as tennis and handball, he finds his skill is dwindling.

Deterioration of Skin

The man's skin begins to sag and wrinkle; the myriad of tiny muscles within the skin gradually lose strength and the skin loses elasticity; in many men, the sebacious (se-bay'-shus) glands reduce their output of oily lubricant and the skin dries. The effects of aging may be particularly severe on the face and hands, where the skin has had most exposure to sun and cold and to physical damage from shaving and manual work.

Skin changes are more likely to be noticed than are some of the other changes (for example, deterioration of the arteries or brittleness of the bones), so those wrinkled hands, bags under the eyes, liver spots, and scar pigmentation can all cause emotional concern quite out of proportion to their real physical importance.

Graying or Loss of Hair

In youth the scalp produces hair and pigments that color it. For some reason in many men (and women, too) the output of coloring matter begins to fail while hair production continues. So hair after hair turns gray. The graying is distributed capriciously: For example, on one man the beard is white while the hair of the head retains its color; another man's head is slate gray and his beard colored. In other men the hair-production system fails first, and the man begins to go bald without turning gray.

We don't know why some men go gray or bald, while others do not. Folklore suggests some connection between hair loss and sexuality, but there are no medical grounds for the belief, other than that the absence of testosterone in women explains the rarity of baldness among them. There is undoubtedly some hereditary pattern at work, because patterns of graying and baldness often pass from father to son. (That, of course, doesn't *explain* the phenomenon; it only shifts the absence of explanation one or more generations into the past.)

Dental Problems

Under primitive living conditions teeth are gradually worn away by chewing; in middle age, the results of this wear become noticeable. However, civilized man's soft food doesn't provide this natural wear. On the contrary, his teeth appear to grow until they are too long for their sockets. The result is receding gums and tooth-neck exposure. Painful defects, or loosening of teeth, are not uncommon by middle age; also, for various reasons, including faulty diet and neglect of tooth cleaning, dental disease takes a further toll.

Some men are so conscious of unsightly tooth defects that they are reluctant to smile. Even if the bad teeth or the gaps are out of sight or even if the man does not care about them, tooth defects still reduce his ability to chew food. Inadequately chewed food cannot be properly digested. Thus, dental problems contribute to the general undermining of the man's health.

Increasing Weight

As he ages, the average man requires less food to maintain health. He is not building new tissue as fast as he did in childhood and adolescence. He is probably using less physical energy than he did as a young man: He has probably given up tennis; he rides instead of walking around the golf course; perhaps he now hires a gardener instead of mowing the lawn and digging the flower beds himself.

But does he therefore eat less? Quite likely, if he has prospered economically, he now consumes *more* rich food and drink than he did before. The inevitable result is an accumulation of fat that makes him look and feel older than he is. Chronic overeating also tends to reduce a man's sexual activity. (With a full belly the natural desire is to rest, or sleep, rather than to undertake exercise.)

Osteoporosis

Osteoporosis—increasing porosity of the bones—is invariably present when the level of androgens (male hormones) is low in a man's system for any long period of time; it is usually absent when androgen levels are normal because androgens are needed to deposit the bone proteins, which in turn allow proper calcium deposition in the man's bone structure. Sex hormones given as therapy for the climacteric are very often effective in curing osteoporosis.

Alcohol Abuse

Excessive alcohol consumption that is continued over several years can directly cause several symptoms of the climacteric; or it will exacerbate other causes that are producing those symptoms.

Of the physical symptoms listed in Chapter 1, chronic alcohol drinking may be a contributory cause of impotence, urinary irregularities, fluid retention, heart symptoms, headaches, and high blood pressure. It may be a major factor in causing and in preventing the cure of peptic ulcers. Continuous, heavy drinking of alcohol causes gastritis: The stomach lining becomes chronically inflamed and swollen and so cannot do its part in digesting food. The man loses his appetite; he sometimes vomits in the morning when his stomach is empty; his tongue is furred; he has frequent headaches and nearly always feels tired; and his desire for sexual activity is reduced.

If one who has drunk heavily does attempt sexual intercourse, he is likely to fail, probably by reason of a weak or short-lasting erection. After a few such disappointing experiences, the man has a permanent fear of failure, leading to a well-established expectation of failure. In such an emotion-laden activity, the expectation of failure produces its own fulfillment; the man becomes afraid to try at all or, if he does try, finds that he has become altogether impotent.

Yet another effect of excessive alcohol drinking is that the liver is gradually converted to scar tissue (cirrhosis of the liver), and its digestive functions become impaired. But the liver has another important function, namely detoxification, the neutralizing of poisons. All men produce a small amount of the female sex hormone estrogen (just as women produce a small amount of the male hormone testosterone). But for the male organism, this estrogen is unwanted and undesirable, and so a healthy liver metabolizes it to get rid of it. A liver damaged by hard drinking cannot do this. The estrogen remains in his body and begins to feminize it. That is the reason why alcoholics frequently develop gynecomastia (gy-ne-ko-mast'-ya), the growth of protuberant breasts like a woman's. They may also get a somewhat feminine distribution of body hair. This partial feminization, too, may expose the man to hurtful remarks from women, remarks that will wound his ego and further impair his virility.

It is well known that an alcoholic tends to become temporarily impotent; but I would emphasize that the impotence produced by persistent, heavy drinking may last long after one has stopped drinking, may even continue for years after one has abandoned the use of alcohol. A woman describes some of the symptoms that alcohol produced in her climacteric husband as "tension, heart attack symptoms, restlessness, irritability, impotence, sweating, rudeness, cruelty (physical and mental)."

Tobacco Smoking

There is some evidence from the Soviet Union and the United States that smoking reduces a man's sex drive. The precise mechanism is not known for certain: it may be because of the toxic effect of nicotine on the autonomic nervous system and the lowering of hormone production.

Headaches

In Chapter 1 I described the tissues of the head that are sensitive to pain. Whatever the initial trigger mechanism, the pain of a headache is caused by swelling (edema) of the tissues or blood vessels, alternate constriction and dilation (pulsation) of blood vessels, or painful muscle contractions.

There are several causes that may bring on one or more of these painful conditions: abnormal handling by the body of salt and water; fluctuating activity of sex hormones; hereditary metabolic abnormalities; physical fatigue, eyestrain, and neck strain; toxins, such as alcohol, caffeine, nicotine, carbon monoxide, and drugs; high blood pressure; hardening of the arteries; impingement of nerve roots by muscle and intervertebral joint strain; and viral or bacterial infections, such as colds, sinusitis, influenza, and meningitis. One or more of these causes can produce cyclical attacks of headache, and obviously the middle-aged man is particularly susceptible to several of them.

Physical Causes of Impotence

For many men impotence will be the most distressing of all the climacteric symptoms. The following is an outline of its principal physical causes:

Abnormalities of the genitals: inborn malformations; abnormalities acquired through infection with venereal disease or other inflammatory disease of the genitals; mutilation by physical injury

Medical conditions: severe cases of diabetes; syphilis; leukemia; alcoholism or drug addiction; extreme hardening of the main artery (the aorta); multiple sclerosis and other diseases of the spinal cord; strokes of a certain type

Surgical conditions: incidental destruction of autonomic nerve fibers in an operation

Brain damage: destruction of certain brain (and spinal cord) centers that are linked to sexual function

Drugs (medical use): hypnotics or tranquilizers, in high or frequent dosage; certain types of antidepressants and antihypertensives

Causes and Effects

It is not hard to see how the physical causes mentioned in this chapter may contribute to the climacteric syndrome. A steady decline of androgen output is eventually going to undermine the man's masculinity.

The man who, because of general physical and emotional decline, always feels weak and tired is never much inclined toward sexual activity; and for men at or above middle age, it is a general rule that the less sex they have, the less they want. (It commonly happens, for example, that middle-aged men whose wives die never seek any other sexual outlet, even after their immediate grief has subsided.)

The man whose skin shows marked signs of aging has perhaps heard some unkind comment about it from a woman, and feels sensitive. The man with gynecomastia may have a similar experience. The man who becomes aware that his hair is graying or falling out may begin to feel old and depressed by the thought of physical deterioration and death. The man who has become very fat certainly finds sexual intercourse more exhausting than when he was younger and slimmer. Perhaps his wife, and other women, find his obesity repulsive and avoid making love with him. Here again, lack of stimulation leads to dwindling of desire. Or perhaps some woman has sneered at his fat paunch, and now he feels reluctant to be seen naked.

Who's to Blame?

We do not at present know why one man's hair should start turning gray in his twenties while another man's keeps its color up into the seventies. We cannot yet say why those 15 percent of men suffer a hormonal decline or why some men's prostate glands enlarge in midlife and other men's do not. But for some of the other symptoms mentioned in this chapter, we can say that the blame lies largely with the man himself; he is paying the price of neglecting his own health. Let us see specifically where he has failed.

Most middle-aged men in the more prosperous parts of the world take too little exercise and eat too much food; moreover, the food they eat is ill-chosen (too rich in animal fats, sugars, and starches), and so, although they are certainly not starving, they suffer from faulty nutrition and nutritional diseases. This faulty nutrition and lack of exercise combine to accelerate and aggravate all the normal changes associated with aging: The muscles, bones, joints, skin, heart, lungs—in fact, all parts of the body—deteriorate sooner than they should.

On top of this many men make excessive use of alcohol, tobacco, and drugs. These poisons would be dangerous enough to a man in otherwise perfect physical condition; they are even more dangerous to a body already weakened by inactivity and poor diet.

Also, many men, even when they recognize that something is wrong with them, are reluctant to see a doctor. (Women generally show more sense about such things.) Even if a man goes to the doctor, he may not frankly say what is bothering him—loss of libido or potency—and may simply mutter something about "feeling run-down." (Many doctors are at fault here. They rarely ask mature patients about their sex lives; a thorough, yet tactful questioning on this subject might reveal some useful information.)

The ordinary man would not hesitate to get his automobile, his television set, or his furnace repaired when necessary. He would not hesitate to tell the serviceman exactly what was wrong. Yet for some reason he won't take the same care of his body. So his physical condition slips from bad to worse, his symptoms are intensified, and he, and his wife, become convinced that he is over the hill.

Some ailments—the common cold and influenza, for example—are self-limited: They last for awhile and then the patient recovers. One may get well faster and more comfortably with treatment, but even without it one recovers anyway. The male climacteric is not like that. It can be considered as a chronic, degenerative ailment that produces unwelcome effects on the sexual, social, and business life of the middle-aged men who experience it. It is not a self-limited or self-corrective disease: Treatment is essential if the man wants to enjoy the rest of his life instead of resigning himself to premature aging and death.

Remission of Symptoms

For the man who is willing to take appropriate action, there are good prospects for remission of symptoms. A fifty-three-year-old who had suffered quite severely from climacteric symptoms undertook a prolonged course of diet and exercise. He reported

> an interesting development: sex desire has been getting much stronger and more frequent in the last two weeks than it had been for years. This may be due to improvement in my general state of health. . . . About all the symptoms remaining are very brief spells of light-headedness (about 30 seconds at a time), and not many of those—plus a little occasional sweating and some mild feelings of heat and chilliness. A fantastic result!

In Chapter 7 I shall offer some detailed suggestions for health improvement that may be expected to produce similar results.

5
Psychological Causes

As far as can be observed, sexual behavior in the lower animals is completely determined by sex hormones and by the lower centers of the brain; in the higher mammals, including man, the higher centers of the brain are actively involved in sexual function. (This is not to minimize the importance of the physical contribution to successful sexual activity.)

Indeed, the whole process of courtship can aptly be compared with the conduct of a political campaign. The would-be candidate must win a nomination; then he may have to fight a primary election, draft a platform, raise funds, compose publicity material, make speeches, shake hands, ingratiate allies, rebut criticism, and always project the desired image of sincerity and dynamism. One false gesture, one inept phrase, can undo all the rest of the good work and lead to defeat.

In Chapter 1 I described the psychosomatic (mind-body) relationship. Here I shall mention a number of psychosomatic factors of the male climacteric.

PEAKS AND VALLEYS

By the time a man reaches middle age, he probably has well-established habits of thinking and feeling that have served as major influences in shaping his life, including his sex life. These habits *can* be changed, of course: One sometimes sees radical transformations under the influence of religion, for example. Yet, in most cases, there are not likely to be any such changes: As the man is at forty or fifty, so he will be till he dies.

Now suppose a man suddenly realizes that he has become, mentally and emotionally, an agglomeration of habits. He has for years nursed hopes of great achievements; he suddenly sees that, if he goes on as he is, there will be no great achievements. He is deep in a rut; he is over the hill, and on the downward slope to the grave.

One man reports "a dissatisfaction with present job, a lament for missed opportunities." Another speaks of "depression, lack of confidence in my own abilities and others, sense of futility with life, a strong cynicism combined with extreme restlessness—generally a strong feeling of dissatisfaction with my life and the way I was living—although I could not determine what I was actually dissatisfied with."

Such painful realizations may be triggered by an outward event. The last child leaves home, for marriage or career. A marriage that has been closely child-centered now requires a thorough reassessment; the father may find he has no meaningful life of his own, nothing of importance left to live for. The mirror, the wife, a photograph, or a friend tells him that his hair is noticeably graying or falling out.

The book of Ecclesiastes (1:2 and 2:22–23) vividly expresses the feelings of the depressed climacteric male: "Vanity of vanities, saith the Preacher . . . all is vanity. . . . For what hath man of all his labour, and of the vexation of his heart, wherein he hath laboured under the sun? For all his days are sorrows, and his travail grief; yea, his heart taketh not rest in the night. This is also vanity." After a long passage of such repinings, the Preacher suddenly switches to a tone of ebullient optimism: "Behold that which I have seen: it is good and comely for one to eat and to drink, and to enjoy the good of all his labour that he taketh under the sun all the days of his life which God giveth him: for it is his portion" (Eccles. 5:18). Such alternations of mood are not uncommon in the climacteric male.

IMPOTENCE AND ITS CAUSES

Without doubt impotence or a serious decline of potency is for many men the most distressing of all the symptoms of the climacteric. (It has even driven some men to suicide.) Let us look at the psychological causes that may bring on this condition. These causes, we may safely say, are widely operative. Dr. Wilhelm Stekel, a disciple of Sigmund Freud, himself psychoanalyzed more than 10,000 patients; he estimated during the 1920s and early 1930s that less than half of all civilized men have what he called "normal potency."

Fear

The man at climacteric may be subject to a variety of fears, some of them newly generated by the changing circumstances of his life, some of them long-repressed and now emerging into consciousness.

FEAR OF AGING

Fear of aging, although perhaps not so well recognized among men as among women, is nevertheless quite common among men. Average life expectancy for males in the United States is now between sixty-seven and sixty-eight years; so the average man's life is half spent when he reaches the age of thirty-four. We don't like to face that fact: to dodge it, we customarily refer to the years between forty-five and sixty as "middle age." (I use the phrase with that meaning here because that is how it is usually understood.)

Subconsciously afraid of age, some men won't face the fact that they are aging. Yet, sooner or later, that fact is forced into consciousness. Perhaps it happens the first time a man hears himself referred to as "middle-aged." Whatever the occasion, it is a severe shock. "Middle-aged! I've got less time to live than I've lived already!"

He reviews his past life, the time when he was at the peak of strength and ambition. Probably he feels disappointed at what he sees—great aspirations, mediocre achievements. He looks to the future, a period of dwindling strength, lost illusions, and so little time left! Will he be able to change gears, to make the rest of his life more smooth-rolling, more productive? He thinks not. No wonder he feels afraid!

It would be easier if he could talk over his fears. Yet in many cases the man is emotionally isolated: He cannot share with his wife, children, or friends the fears that beset him. He would like to be comforted but does not like to admit to what might be considered a weak emotional state.

He engages in sexual fantasies, yet never dares to talk about them or to put them into practice. Perhaps he could do so with younger people but not with his contemporaries, who are less broad-minded. "What would people think of *that*," he worries, "in a man of my age?"

He may have picked up some erroneous ideas about the aging process and the mental and physical, especially sexual, changes that he may expect. The most dangerous error, from our point of view, is the notion that using his sexual powers is going to wear them out. In Chapter 4 I pointed out the falsity of this notion.

Thus, if fear of aging makes the man do less, the fear becomes self-fulfilling. He finds that his potency dwindles or disappears altogether.

FEAR OF WOMEN

A man may be secretly afraid of the vastly greater sexual capability of women. Tests under clinical conditions have shown some women capable of six orgasms in thirty minutes and more than fifty in one night. A man at the peak of his sexual power is doing well if he attains three to five orgasms in one night. Some men, perhaps unconsciously, choose to marry frigid women who will not shame them by making demands that they could not fulfill.

The increasing use of effective methods of birth control, together with the recent reassessment of the whole male-female relationship, has tended to give women much more freedom in expressing their sexuality. Many women who seemed to be frigid are beginning to demand sexual satisfaction; if they cannot get it from their husbands, they may go elsewhere.

Another possibility is that, when the last child is grown and off her hands, the wife may gladly drop her long-played role as mother and homemaker and begin to shape a new life as a free, independent woman, returning to a former career or taking up a new one. This upheaval alone can be emotionally disturbing to a husband; it undermines his position as economic anchor of the family. But the wife's new job may produce sharp changes in her character: She is meeting new women and men, absorbing new ideas about her function as an economic, social, and sexual being. The husband may well find this new-model wife rather frightening. He fears what she may think or say to him or what she may tell their friends if he cannot meet her sexual demands, if he fails in the "numbers game." And of course his fear of failure increases the likelihood of failure.

FEAR OF FATHERHOOD

By the time they reach middle age, many men are tired of fatherhood; they definitely do not want any more children. For such a man the fear of causing pregnancy may be strong enough to make him impotent, even if, intellectually, he knows all about birth control.

FEAR OF VENEREAL DISEASE

A man who is seeking sexual relations with women other than his wife must face the risk of venereal disease, a risk that has been rapidly increasing in recent years. For some men the fear of syphilis or gonorrhea may be enough to produce impotence. If a man knows or suspects that his wife is having sex with other men, he may fear catching venereal disease from her, which may make him impotent.

FEAR OF REJECTION

When a man is making sexual advances to a woman for the first time—especially a woman much younger than himself—he may be afraid that she will reject him, perhaps with some unkind remarks about his age, his figure, his falling hair, and so on. Or he may fear that even if he accomplishes intercourse once, the woman will find his efforts unsatisfying and will reject his requests for a repeat performance. Such fears may be enough to make him impotent.

OEDIPUS COMPLEX

Many psychologists and psychiatrists, particularly those of the Freudian school, believe that in middle age a man with a latent Oedipus complex may suddenly see in his aging wife a frightening resemblance to his own mother as she was when he was in his teens. Such a man may very well have chosen his wife because of a dimly perceived resemblance to the adored mother. But now a subconscious fear of incest may render the man incapable of making love to his wife, despite years of satisfactory lovemaking in the past.

Another man might reject this suddenly repulsive wife-mother by drifting into homosexual circles and so avoiding marital relations. The wife might have difficulty in accepting his new friends.

FEAR OF UNDERACHIEVEMENT

A man may set unrealistically high sexual goals for himself and then become alarmed when he cannot attain them. For example, some men think they should be able to produce a firm erection promptly, whenever they feel it would be convenient. This is *not* by any means always attainable: The occasional failure to do it does *not* necessarily indicate that the man has one foot in the grave.

Boredom

I said in Chapter 2 that in midlife many couples become bored with sex. The idea might have seemed inconceivable to them when they were courting, yet it is true. Let us see how it may happen.

I have gained the impression in marital counseling (and many other authorities would agree) that the typical couple needs about three years to become sexually adjusted to one another. Through a series of trials and errors the sexual pattern becomes established over this three-year period; it changes very little in later years. Few couples seem able to continue experimentation in sexual practices past this time, especially once children have arrived on the scene.

So the couple has established a sexual pattern. Love, which once ruled supreme in the marriage, must now yield precedence to the demands of the children, of the home, and of earning a living. Sexual activities are restricted to certain hours when all other duties have been fulfilled, usually at night, when the kids have settled down to sleep and are not likely to disturb their parents.

Sex becomes one item in a well-established schedule, perhaps with no higher rank than mealtime, viewing television, or going to church. As time goes on, routine degenerates into boredom. After twenty years of the same, oft-repeated sexual activities, the partners tend to lose sight of the need to work at the marital relationship.

Perhaps a domineering husband, insisting on his conjugal rights, makes coitus simply one more chore for his already overburdened wife. He abandons whatever he used to practice in the arts of courtship.

Chronic fatigue in either partner may diminish the desire for and the pleasure of sex, to the point where it is approached as just another duty, like remembering to pay the light bill or the insurance premium. Joy is replaced by boredom; they both begin to wonder what has happened to their romance.

The man who is perceptive enough to notice and wonder about this boredom in his wife may run into a special problem. Perhaps she has read about, or a woman friend or a daughter has told her about, new possibilities for sexual gratification. She mentions the subject to her husband, but he at once goes on the defensive and interprets her remarks as a reflection on his fading physical charms and dwindling sexual powers: "I obviously can't fascinate or satisfy her the way I once did!" He makes a desperate effort to go along with her suggestions, fumbles, fails a few times, and may very well end up impotent.

Another man, beset by this creeping boredom, begins to nurse fantasies about other women, about new sexual experiences, more exciting than any he enjoys at home. He draws the conclusion that his marriage has become a dull dead end in which he is stuck, as the real, exciting sex life goes on outside.

One type of man is likely to feel especially keenly this boredom with wife and sex—the man who married very young. When in midlife he begins to feel new sexual urges, he thinks it is because his early marriage robbed him of what should have been a fun-filled, exciting young manhood. He may lose his head and set out to make up for lost time in the few years that he thinks he has left. He may still be fond of his wife. He doesn't want to hurt her; but he wants to escape from that marriage! He will give generous support to her and the children, but he can scarcely wait to get out of the house and start living it up.

No More Children

I said earlier that for some men, fear of fathering a child was capable of producing impotence. For other men a contrary emotion is operative. A man may react strongly to his wife's menopause, to the knowledge that he will never father another child, at least with her. An unmarried man may undergo a similar shock when he accepts the fact that he probably will never father a child at all.

I said in Chapter 1 that there is usually no physical relationship between fertility—the ability to produce living sperm—and potency—the penile ability to conduct sexual intercourse. But there may sometimes be an important psychological relationship.

Suppose a man discovers that he is sterile or that he has so low a sperm count as to give practically no chance of fathering a child. For some men this would be a delightful surprise: They get the benefit of a vasectomy without the expense. For others it is a severe emotional shock: They feel they have been demanned; they become impotent.

I heard of a case where a man in his mid-twenties, sexually active, discovered in the course of a routine medical examination that he would never be able to father a child. Within two weeks he had experienced a complete character change, becoming a puritanical religious fanatic, an absolute pest to his old friends.

Whatever the basis, the realization that one cannot reproduce is, for many men, a shock capable of triggering a galaxy of symptoms, including impotence.

The Will to Impotence

Some men develop a subconscious "will to impotence," which may be caused by a desire to escape from the responsibilities of being a husband and father. Or it may be a retaliation against a domineering or overly demanding wife. These men can often be temporarily cured by the placebo effect of a pseudoaphrodisiac.

Mutilation Complex

Some men develop an exaggerated idea of the effects of injuries they have suffered or of surgery they have undergone. For example, vasectomies or most prostate operations should not in any way impair the patient's sexual performance; yet some men become impotent afterwards. They *think* their sexual powers have been destroyed, and their thoughts become realities.

Guilt Feelings

The autonomic nervous system, although beyond the direct control of the will, is nevertheless very sensitive to emotional stimulation. A man can, for example, aid the erecting mechanism of his penis by deliberately conjuring up some sexually stimulating thought (a striptease act seen the night before, for example). Conversely, he can obstruct the mechanism by nursing feelings of fear or guilt. For example, if the man lets himself dwell on such thoughts as "I'm betraying my wife," or "She trusts me, but I'm not worthy of her trust," and so on, then he is likely to become impotent with his wife, no matter how well he may perform with another woman.

Feelings of guilt about spending too much time and thought on work, politics, sports, and so on, and too little on their wives might for some men be sufficient to produce either temporary or permanent impotence.

Any kind of sexual difficulty or failure will, for many men, arouse guilt feelings even where, in terms of the law, or of commonly accepted moral standards, no real guilt is involved. Such men feel a moral responsibility to give a brilliant sexual performance every time that their wives want it. When they fail, as most men sometimes do, these sexual perfectionists feel morbidly guilty, and this guilt increases the chance of further failures.

It is because of this guilt feeling that many men will not consult the doctor about their climacteric problems. The wives do not share the guilt, so they go to the doctor instead.

Sterilization

Increasing numbers of men and women are choosing sterilization as a safe, certain, convenient means of birth control. It is possible that because of their religious beliefs or other reasons, some people might be afraid of having guilt feelings after the operation. However, in recent studies in Canada no feelings of guilt among the men or women involved were admitted or reported.

LOST LIBIDO

I have so far been discussing mainly the causes of impotence. Another common problem at the climacteric is loss of libido. It is to be expected that as a man ages, he should experience a slight, gradual reduction of libido; but any substantial, rapid decrease of libido is a sign of the climacteric.

Libido—the desire for sexual activity—is aroused not only by the immediate sight of a sexually attractive woman: It depends largely on frequent stimulation by erotic memories and fantasies. The richer one's treasure chest of pleasurable sex memories, and the more often one looks into it, the stronger and longer-lasting will be one's sex drive. Unfortunately for many men, the treasure chest is not very richly stocked, and as the years go by, it is more and more rarely opened.

I have already mentioned the morning erection as evidence of sexually oriented dreams; the pity is that most of these dreams are so soon forgotten and that for so many men nocturnal sex fantasies are never carried over into the waking hours, when they would do more good.

By middle age many men have developed a grim, earnest attitude toward life: They think there would be something immature, something demeaning, in spending time on sex memories and fantasies. They neglect, or avoid, any stimulation by women or by sex-oriented books, films, magazines, and so on.

Such absence of stimulation will tend to weaken a man's libido; then he comes to believe, falsely, that he is sexually worn out, finished.

STRESS

Emotional stress can produce a great variety of physical effects on the person who suffers it. Long before orthodox medicine took much notice of the subject, it was vividly expressed in common speech: "You're breaking my heart." "I can't stomach that." "This breaks me up." "He gripes me." "She makes me sick."

In particular, stress can upset the operation of the sexual system: For example, a sudden fright may cause a sexually aroused man abruptly to lose his erection. Prolonged stress—fear, guilt, shame, illness, exhaustion, for example—may cause a long-lasting reduction in the activity of the whole sexual system, a dwindling of sexual desire, a loss of erectile ability, and a diminution of testosterone and sperm production.

Emotional stress, intellectual overactivity, and fatigue can cause headaches, pseudoangina, depression, and several other of the nonsexual symptoms of the climacteric. Emotional stress, especially if it is prolonged, often drives men to seek relief in the excessive use of alcohol or in drugs. I have described elsewhere the deleterious effects of alcohol and drugs on the sexual system.

SEXUAL DEVIATIONS

Men who turn to homosexuality or other deviations from their normal activity at the climacteric have not suddenly developed a new sexuality: They have begun to manifest long-established tendencies.

Most adolescents have some homosexual feelings. For many of them the tendency passes off without ever leading to any action; for others, a period of homosexual activity is eventually superseded by a strengthening interest in girls. The young man camouflages, or perhaps completely forgets, what he now considers to have been a temporary deviation and for twenty years or more presents an effective heterosexual image.

Nevertheless, at the climacteric some heterosexuals experience a revival of that long-repressed homosexuality. Richard M., a married man, had a friend, H., who was a homosexual. M. sometimes wondered why H. seemed to work so hard at maintaining the friendship; yet H. was a congenial man, so they continued it for several years.

M.'s marriage broke up and he left his wife. Soon afterward, H. made an advance: "Richard, did you ever think of yourself as a potential homosexual?" Richard rebuffed him and eventually remarried; yet he commented, "If I had had some leanings toward homosexuality, that was the time, when I was feeling depressed and lonely, that I might have accepted H.'s proposition."

DUALISM

In Chapter 1 I mentioned the theory that sees man as made up of two entities: mind and matter, or soul and body, temporarily associated. For Plato there was no question which of the two should be in control: "The soul of man is immortal and imperishable." Sallust said, "The soul is the captain and ruler of the life of mortals." Descartes said, "I think, therefore I am." In his *Essay on Man* Alexander Pope expresses the dualist theory but seems not to know which is superior. He describes man as

> In doubt to deem himself a God or Beast;
> In doubt his mind or body to prefer.

In *Song of Myself* Walt Whitman goes a step further:

> I have said that the soul is not more than the body
> And I have said that the body is not more than the soul.

The dualist view of man has lingered in medical practice: Until recently physicians concerned themselves with man's body as a machine more or less independent of his mind or consciousness. The patient was ready to accept this theory, to assume that the machine was at fault and not himself—his mind or spirit. Many present-day patients fight against accepting the concept of emotionally induced illness: They feel that this somehow carries a burden of guilt or failure, as of a captain who had navigated carelessly and wrecked his ship. Such guilt feelings are reinforced by the well-meant advice of friends and relatives: "Control yourself. Pull yourself together." They do not consider who is supposed to be controlling whom; they do not ask who is pulling, and what is being pulled.

This chapter has demonstrated that mind and body are *not* separate entities, that the mind must be continually affecting the body, and vice versa. Failure to understand and accept this connection will in fact be a major cause of physical and mental ill-health. In Chapter 8 I shall offer some suggestions for reaching this understanding and acceptance.

THE STIFF UPPER LIP

A major psychological problem in our society is the convention that men do not admit weakness, do not complain, and certainly never weep. A spell of loud sobbing, a copious flow of tears, can provide excellent therapy for fear, grief, remorse, anger—for a whole galaxy of unpleasant emotions. Yet this therapy is not available for the ordinary man: Tears would be regarded, by him and by his friends, as a sign of disgraceful, unmanly weakness. For the same reason a man is less likely than a woman to consult psychologists or marriage counselors for aid in the face of sexual problems. His masculine ego would feel ashamed to confess, even to a stranger, that he is lacking in libido or potency.

A nonsexual example of the same attitude is the man who refuses to accept the back troubles that are common in middle age: He will insist that the pain and stiffness are caused not by a normal aging process but by "sitting in a draft" or some such mischance. The man gets no treatment, and his sore back remains a lasting handicap in his work, his leisure, and his sex life.

The need to work so hard at being "manly," then, is a major psychological cause for many of the symptoms of the climacteric.

6

Social Causes

All men are influenced to some degree by outside forces, such as religion, tradition, television, newspapers, advertising, family, and friends. Even the most stubborn individualist cannot escape them. The boy's mind is molded by his peers and the educational system under which he grows up. The man's life is shaped by the work he does, by the woman he marries, and by his political affiliations. For many men social acceptance and economic security depend upon the goodwill of their associates; to maintain that goodwill they conform to community standards.

Most important for our purpose is the fact that as such forces influence a man's beliefs and conduct, they influence his physical and mental health, shape his sexual attitudes and behavior, and help determine whether his sex life is to be short or long, frustrating or satisfying.

WORK

For many middle-aged men, work has become the most important element in their lives—more important than wife, children, religion, or recreation. It is no wonder that what happens at work can in many ways hasten the onset of the male climacteric.

Boredom and Dissatisfaction with Work

Many men are doing routine, noncreative work that they feel is beneath them, that does not give scope to their abilities. They are continually bored. There are men whose work might be considered by others as being creative and enjoyable; yet even for some of them there comes a time when the interest has evaporated.

Alexander Damon, the architect in Taylor Caldwell's *The Listener*, says, "What meaning is there, for anyone. . . . For what is a man born? To throw up more and more buildings, more and more offices, more and more apartment houses? For what? Tell me, in God's name, for what? . . . All is repetition, a treadmill, a squirrel cage. No matter what you do! Nothing has any lasting meaning, significance, worth."*

In Alexander Damon, Taylor Caldwell vividly depicts a man at the climacteric. In his mid-forties, he sometimes has fits of irrational anger and at other times long spells of depression, inertia, and apathy; he is about to divorce his third wife. He is undergoing psychoanalysis but seems to have derived no benefit from it; and he is an alcoholic.

Then there are men who don't particularly dislike their work but cannot stand the people they have to work with, perhaps they would be happier working for themselves but have never dared to try it.

Consider the case of the man who for the first twenty or thirty years of his career has been kept going by hope—hope of technical accomplishment, hope of promotion, hope of power, hope of wealth. Then one day he finds that his hopes have evaporated. Perhaps it is the retirement of a colleague who had seemed not much older than himself and who has now gone without achieving much; perhaps it is the promotion of a younger man over his head; perhaps it is the growing pressure of women on what had been a male preserve. Whatever the reason, he has lost hope, and work suddenly seems less interesting, less satisfying. One such man describes the change:

> The most profound change was toward work. I realized that perhaps my entire past business career was simply a waste of

* Quoted by permission from Taylor Caldwell, *The Listener* copyright © 1960 by Reback & Reback; published by Doubleday & Company, Inc.

time. This resulted in my attitude to the growth ethic and "selling" of competitive free enterprise being changed. I realized what a vast make-work swindle the whole marketing apparatus was. I began to research and write a book about the subject, but as I researched the angrier I became, and the more critical the book became. The book effectively ended my career in the business world. . . . Was there an unconscious "burning of bridges" in that development? It's impossible for me to know objectively, but in the transitional stage my business colleagues knew something had happened to me. I began defending *the consumer* at board meetings and conferences. I talked about ethics and business responsibility. I was quite literally shunned and avoided toward the end, and it was a relief to my boss when I finally quit, I'm sure.

Occupational Stress and Sex

For several climacteric symptoms, we find that the most significant causative factor is occupational stress. An instructive comparison can be drawn between work and war. Every veteran knows how low a man's libido sinks as he nears the front line: The survival instinct overrules the mating instinct. The fighting man's sex drive is usually not restored until he withdraws to safer territory. And so for many men, work is a merciless battle for survival: The man who cannot or will not fight fiercely enough goes under. Uncertainty of the future and fear of not surviving the contest frighten the middle-aged man more than the young beginner. Vocational battle fatigue may drive the climacteric male to the breaking point.

The relationship between economic potency and sexual potency is, psychologically speaking, an intimate one. Both are commonly looked upon as a measure of virility; this idea probably goes back to preagrarian forms of society in which the best hunter was the best provider and the most desirable mate. For such men an economic downturn, or just the fear of it, may lead to a downturn of sexual desire and sexual potency.

A man described his "awareness of economic vulnerability,

especially during the last few years when promotions might be slow, although income may be higher than ever." A woman reported that her husband rarely had a sexual urge and even then had difficulty in carrying out intercourse. She noticed that business problems would trigger spells of physical symptoms.

Zoo operators have long been aware that the mating habits of animals change—in some cases mating ceases altogether—when they are held in captivity. The same disturbance of mating habits may occur in men who feel they are being held captive by social and economic forces beyond their control.

I said above that economic stress may impair a man's virility. There is another interesting connection. Suppose a man's erotic potency fails him through some other cause while he still remains economically successful: Then he may try to retain his wife's affection by showering her with material goods, such as furs, jewels, big cars, and costly vacations.

Occupational Stress and Other Symptoms

Peptic ulcers and coronary artery disease have sometimes been called "managers' diseases," yet they may be found in men who are suffering stress and nervous tension anywhere on the vocational ladder. (Indeed, ulcers are practically unknown among men who are free from such stress and tension.) Middle-aged men are particularly vulnerable. They must face the competition of younger men; their energy reserves are less than those of younger men; and they cannot adjust so easily as younger men to technical and social changes.

Understandably, these stresses stir up negative emotions, such as fear, anger, frustration, guilt, and feelings of inadequacy and rejection. These emotions can upset the autonomic nervous system, particularly the vagus nerve, an important part of the parasympathetic system, which controls the digestive organs. To put the effect in simple terms, the man's digestive system is overstimulated to the point where it begins to turn against itself: Excess acid eats away at the walls of esophagus, stomach, or duodenum to form ulcers.

Stress has been found to give captive animals peptic ulcers, particularly in zoos that are overcrowded; yet that "captive feeling" and overcrowding are only two of many harmful factors that are at work on men. The kind of men who get ulcers commonly have acquired habits that tend to worsen the condition, habits such as irregular timing of eating, eating too quickly, skipping meals, frequent choice of coarse, acidic, fried, and spicy foods, talking of worrisome subjects at the table, excessive drinking of coffee and alcohol, and excessive smoking.

Yet I would emphasize that simply changing your eating and drinking habits is no cure. As the saying goes, "It's not what you eat, but what's eating you, that causes your ulcers." I shall offer in Chapters 7 and 8 some specific suggestions for ulcer victims and their families.

Another stress-induced disease often found among zoo amimals is arteriosclerosis (hardening of the arteries), a condition that is practically unknown among animals in the wild state. Stress will produce the same disease in men.

Excessive Involvement with Work

Work produces undesirable effects not only on those men who are dissatisfied with, anxious about, or failing at their work but also on some of those who are happy and successful. Some middle-aged men, especially successful professional and business men, are, as the saying goes, married to their jobs: Work gives them the emotional fulfillment that some other men receive from their wives.

Often the reason may be loss of sexual potency: The man stays away from the conjugal bed to prevent his wife from finding out; or perhaps he feels better if he can prove his "economic manhood" in the marketplace. Some other men have a different motive. They feel they must fulfill the expectations of their friends and business associates, must live up to whatever is the public image of their particular line of business: "A doctor can't drive a Volkswagen!" "You've *never* been to Hawaii?" "You really should play the stock market." "You mean to say you don't play golf?"

Even one's amusements, by this job-based standard, have to be representative, and preferably competitive.

The drive for compliance in these side issues, however exciting and enjoyable, leads to increased expenditure of time and strength on work and leaves less time and strength for home, family, and sex life. A woman reported that she has observed in her husband and some of their male friends a concern for careers and reassessment of their goals: "Am I working too hard and not enjoying life enough?" A man, successful and genuinely happy in his work, may still sometimes ask himself such questions and may feel depressed when he finds the answer is "Maybe" or "Yes."

Fatigue

The man who is chronically exhausted—for example, from anxiety, overwork, or lack of sleep—may become impotent. (A well-known example, even among young men, is wedding-night impotence: The bridegroom is physically and emotionally worn out from prewedding preparations and parties, the ceremony, the reception, and a tiring drive to the honeymoon site.) Middle-aged men who endure two hours' freeway driving plus seven hours' work for five days a week may be in such a state of chronic exhaustion that they go for months without ever getting an erection.

Retirement

For a man who dislikes his work, retirement is something to look forward to. But what about the man for whom work is enjoyable and important? How does he feel when suddenly he faces the specter of compulsory retirement?

He has to know about retirement regulations, of course; but he thought of them only as applying to other men—older men. Now he suddenly realizes that his own working life is considerably more than half over; he begins to wonder what he will do when he has no work to do, how long he will live after retirement.

Sixty-five is, for many men, a needlessly early retirement age: They could still do years of good work. Yet there is a developing tendency to force retirement upon men of sixty or even younger. Moreover, the trend to earlier, compulsory retirement makes it difficult for unemployed men above forty or forty-five to find work. The employer thinks, "We won't get enough out of this guy to recover the cost of training him before we have to start paying him a pension. Better hire someone younger."

Many physicians have noticed that the morbidity rate (the incidence of sickness) in men increases with retirement; there is a particularly sharp increase in mental and emotional disorders. About a year after retirement, the death rate for men increases steeply, including a sharp rise in suicides. One physician who had a general practice in a West Coast retirement area said,

> I see it happen over and over again. A prairie farmer sells his farm, moves out here to the coast and buys a condominium. The first week, he's busy helping his wife fix up the apartment. The second week he's looking over the beach and park, loafing around, admiring the view. The third week, he's in my office, complaining of mysterious pains in his chest.

So the middle-aged man has good reason to fear early retirement.

WOMEN

As I said in Chapter 1, changes in a man's relationship with women may be among the most conspicuous symptoms of the climacteric; they can also be among its most important causes.

Negative Conditioning

A young man's original enthusiastic attitude toward women and sex may be radically changed during courtship and marriage. His sweetheart makes him feel that her condescending to his frequent sexual demands ought to be rewarded by gifts, by yielding to her will, and by doing things to please her or by refraining from acts or actions that might displease her. If he annoys her, she can enforce his dependence, or punish him, by withholding sex. (In the classical Greek play *Lysistrata* a war between Sparta and Athens was stopped through the withholding of sex by the angry warriors' wives.)

After marriage the wife continues the same tactics. So the man finds his sex drive repeatedly frustrated: And frustration is a potent means of reducing and eventually destroying the sex drive. Some oversensitive men may feel hesitant to request intercourse because it seems such an imposition on the less-interested wife.

Some young men do not have an enthusiastic attitude toward sex. They were taught by their mothers to think of sex as "dirty." The mother may have caught him masturbating, telling him how naughty he is and warning him, "God is watching you all the time." Some victims of this sort of conditioning are later helped by girl friends and wives to a better attitude. Some unlucky ones get wives who reinforce the connection of sex with dirt. These men end up feeling guilty about their sex drives and sexual acts; and this guilt is as effective as frustration in reducing and destroying the sex drive.

A woman can symbolically emasculate a man by overtaxing his earning power which, as I said earlier, often symbolizes his sexual power. Sexually frustrated wives and divorcées sometimes use this weapon.

Changing Social Attitudes

There is much talk in present-day society of the new sexual freedom and its supposed benefits. (One of the "benefits" is the skyrocketing incidence of venereal disease among teen-agers.) A middle-aged man who married young and who never enjoyed that sexual freedom may wonder what he missed. He may think, "I should be catching up on the fun I missed as a young single man." Yet he may be afraid to try for fear of failure or for fear of being laughed at.

One man said, "Everything around you is changing fast: people, buildings, values, cultural exchanges, sexual mores, religious feelings. . . . It's like standing on quicksand with weights tied to each shoe. You're too old to change—too rigid and tied to tradition to make the move that might free you."

Sex Taboos

A taboo is sometimes thought of as a quaint custom prevalent only among primitive peoples. In reality, a taboo is a powerful force controlling the behavior and affecting the mental and emotional health of a large part of present-day urbanized, mechanized society. Important for our purpose are taboos about sex and the aging man.

SEX IS FOR REPRODUCTION ONLY

One taboo, long-established in the Christian tradition, prescribes that sexual intercourse is to be performed only for the purpose of begetting children. The sex organs are referred to as "generative organs." Sexual pleasure—if one ever experiences it—is considered to be merely a by-product, a reward for doing one's procreative duty; it is certainly not to serve as a motive for any kind of sexual activity.

Saint Augustine, the theologian and Christian bishop who flourished at the time of the fall of the Roman Empire, was an influential exponent of this concept. His book *The City of God* (begun in A.D. 412) devotes several chapters to the "evil of lust" and "sexual uncleanness." He laments that it is not possible to beget children without "this lust"; he says it is appropriate that the sex organs are called "shameful."

The dualistic concept of the inferiority and earthy, animal nature of the human body gave rise to this taboo. Even today we often hear such expressions as the following: "It's the animal in me that loves sex." "My body craves for sex, in spite of myself." "The animal in me gets the better of me."

For more than fifteen centuries the belief survived in some sections of the Christian church that even between married couples sexual relations were somehow wicked and that children were begotten "in sin."

I recall the case of a Hutterite couple. The husband was a very pious man from a family of strict believers; after he had fathered all the children he wanted, he considered it sinful to continue sex relations. He suffered greatly from this self-imposed abstinence but continued it for fear of damnation. The wife, too, was deeply disturbed by his behavior because he had been a very affectionate husband and an excellent lover. After a few years, the stress of this sexless life broke up the marriage.

The Peace Mission Movement, established in the United States in the 1920s, prescribed an even more austere regime. Its founder and leader, Father Divine, completely forbade sexual intercourse for his followers. He set the example with his second wife—a woman about fifty years younger than himself—who remained a virgin throughout their married life.

The sex-is-sinful theory was, at least to some degree, repudiated by the second Vatican Ecumenical Council, 1963–65, which issued a public statement that the conjugal sex act is "noble and worthy" and that it "promotes that mutual self-giving by which spouses enrich each other with a joyful and thankful will." It remains to be seen how many of the Protestant sects will modify or abolish their sex taboos.

Meanwhile, many men are affected by these taboos. For the man to whom sexual pleasure is sinful, the effort of conducting intercourse and the experience of orgasm can become tiresome, even disgusting—much like a spell of diarrhea. He is likely to welcome any physical changes in midlife that diminish his sex drive; he will probably take the first opportunity to cease his sexual activity altogether.

GRANDPARENTS DON'T HAVE SEX

The taboo against elderly people having sex springs in part from the one previously mentioned: The implication is that people past the reproductive age should not bother with sex any longer because it has become a sterile activity, disgusting and selfish. "What would the grandchildren think?" expresses the guilt feelings associated with sex between grandparents.

At one time there was, perhaps, a reason for this taboo: The risk of producing defective children increases rapidly as a woman approaches the age of grandmotherhood. So it was to the interest of society that couples of this age should cease to have children; the way to ensure that was to discourage them from having sexual intercourse. But for people who practice birth control, the taboo has no purpose. Many grandparents nowadays disregard it and enjoy themselves, no matter what the kids think or say.

Yet many do not. Many men become grandfathers just at the age when they might be susceptible to the climacteric. Some of these men, although their physical capability remains undiminished, are affected, consciously or unconsciously, by the taboo. They begin to feel guilt about sex; they enjoy it less, practice it less frequently, or give it up altogether.

NO WIFE, NO SEX

Men who lose their wives in middle age or later may understandably suffer a temporary loss of libido. However, after the worst of the grief has passed, sex drive will often return. For such a man sex life will be determined in part by the attitudes toward sex prevalent in the society in which he lives. In some cultures middle-aged and old men have ready access to young women for sexual activity; in our society, as a general rule, they do not.

Many men in this situation might be willing to defy the opinions of their friends and look for young girl friends. Yet they feel self-conscious about the fact that they are not so attractive physically as they were twenty-five years earlier. Such men will often pretend to have lost interest in women; by not seeking any new sexual contact, they avoid the risk of a humiliating rebuff.

Such an excuse will be readily accepted by a man's family and friends. There is a common belief that, somewhere in his forties or fifties, a man should expect to suffer a marked decline in his sexual desires and sexual abilities. Indeed, the middle-aged man who still seeks a full, vigorous sex life is, in the eyes of many people, a disgusting figure.

Here, too, there may once have been good grounds for such a taboo. In some societies, a high maternal death rate would produce a considerable surplus of men over women. It was obviously desirable in such a society that the older men should leave the available women for the younger men. But in times like ours, when women outnumber men, this taboo, too, has no purpose.

MASTURBATION IS DANGEROUS

There is reason to believe that a great number of aging men take to masturbation, or masturbate more than they used to, as a means of sexual satisfaction. There are several common reasons for this.

First, a man and wife have become bored with marital sex relations; they have intercourse more and more infrequently. They do not know about, or perhaps do not like to try, techniques that might revitalize their sex life. The man's sex drive is not satisfied on such meager rations, so he finds relief through masturbation.

Second, for one reason or another—illness or quarreling, for example—a man cannot have any sex relations with his wife. He does not want to break up the marriage altogether, but he has to get sexual satisfaction somehow.

Third, a man has no sex partner and does not want to take the trouble of looking for one. Masturbation is the easy way out.

Whatever the reason it is used, masturbation serves the purpose very well for the man who can enjoy it; yet, because of the taboo, many men have grave doubts and fears about practicing it.

In most societies masturbation by girls and women seems to have been tolerated as harmless; perhaps that is because, no matter how often a woman masturbates, it does not lessen her reproductive ability. For men, on the other hand, nearly all the great religions have strictly forbidden masturbation. Obviously, after successfully masturbating, a man is, for a longer or shorter time (depending on his current state of virility), delayed from resuming sexual intercourse; moreover, there was a widespread notion that each man had only a limited supply of semen and that his sacred duty was to save it for procreation.

The Bible tells (Gen. 38:9) how the Lord slew Onan the masturbator for his sin. (Many writers, as if to emphasize the serious nature of the "offense," have referred to masturbation as onanism.) Even for an involuntary ejaculation a man was considered unclean and had to undergo a ritual purification of his body and clothes (Lev. 15:16–17).

Even among people who have no such religious beliefs, there survives a mass of frightening folklore about the supposed effects of masturbation—deterioration of the brain or spinal cord, mental illness, blindness, uncontrollable trembling of the hands, inability to look other people in the eye, and so on. There is also the notion that, quite apart from its supposed moral and physical dangers, masturbation is a childish pastime, and for that reason alone a grown man should be ashamed of doing it.

In fact, there is no evidence that masturbation does the slightest harm, physically or mentally, to those who practice it. Yet, although masturbation itself is a harmless pleasure, the guilt and fear associated with it may in some cases lead to chronic anxiety states or psychosomatic illnesses. In this way the middle-aged man who for one reason or another is regularly masturbating may induce some of the symptoms of the climacteric.

HOMOSEXUALITY IS SINFUL

Active homosexuals are violating several taboos, among which are the following: Sexual activity is for reproduction only, and obviously homosexuals are not going to reproduce themselves; there is only one "right" sexual act (penetration of the vagina by the penis) and only one "right" position for its performance (horizontal, with the man uppermost); sexual pleasure for its own sake is undesirable, even sinful; and sexual activity is permissible only for married male-female couples.

As I mentioned in Chapter 5, some middle-aged men experience a revival of long-dormant homosexual interests. Some may become practicing homosexuals and at the same time feel guilty about it; others who do not practice may feel the same guilt for having the "forbidden" desire. Persistent guilt feelings may well help to produce some of the symptoms of the climacteric.

NAKEDNESS IS SINFUL

In our society this taboo has lately been weakened among youngsters, but for many older people it remains in full force—particularly objectionable for them would be the sight of the sexual organs. Many middle-aged men have never seen their wives naked. Husbands and wives undress separately; for bed, they wear form-concealing pajamas and nightgowns. They make love in the dark to avoid the forbidden sight of each other's bodies. Never having achieved the maximum pleasure from sex, they will be that much readier to renounce it if some physical or emotional difficulty should arise.

A modified form of the taboo asserts that the aging body, male or female, is especially unfit to be seen, that it is repulsive and incapable of giving or experiencing sexual pleasure. Men who accept this taboo will tend, in midlife, to lose the desire, perhaps even the ability, for sexual activity.

ODOR TABOOS

There is a widespread belief that the natural odors of the body and breath are repulsive. The large sale of deodorants, perfumes, scented toothpastes, and mouthwashes testifies to the force of this taboo. The believer in this taboo is more or less nervous of being physically close to another person.

Second Marriages

Suppose a middle-aged man, after the death of his wife or after a divorce, remarries. It is quite likely that he will take a woman considerably younger than his first wife—perhaps a woman young enough to be his own daughter. The young bride wins at one stroke a financial and social position that a husband of her own age group could not have offered her. For the man, it is an ego-inflating situation to have the world believe that he can satisfy the erotic needs of his beautiful young wife.

But the bridegroom faces a number of difficulties. I will not discuss here such questions as alimony, criticism from relatives and in-laws, and jealousy from his children by his first wife: He would have to face those, no matter whom he married. I will deal with the problems that arise specifically from the gap in age between him and his new wife.

In the first place, it is rare to find a middle-aged man who can keep up physically with a woman fifteen or twenty years his junior. At tennis, swimming, skiing, climbing, and dancing, she can probably outperform and outlast him; if she does not do so, the man will sooner or later wonder whether she is holding back to spare his feelings. In bed the same thing applies. Alexander Pope, in *January and May*, tells of the knight who took a young wife. Within a week, the bride was lying miserably awake while

The lumpish husband snored away the night,
Till coughs awaked him near the morning light.

Even suppose that the husband is exceptionally fit and for some time can equal the young wife in physical activities and in sex: How long can it continue—two years, five years, ten years?

These difficulties will not apply to all marriages. Indeed, many of these May–December marriages turn out very well. But one problem is unavoidable: An age difference of fifteen or twenty years means that there is a vast difference in social, economic, cultural and political values. Such differences cause enough trouble between parents and children, where we expect them, where they develop gradually, and where parental love helps to bridge them: They are much more troublesome between a bride and groom who have no common family background and perhaps do not even know each other very well, as many second marriages are hasty.

There are likely to be noticeable differences in sexual attitudes, too. The older man has grown up in what his young wife would regard as a puritanical era. She has acquired her sexual standards from a time when sexual knowledge is widely disseminated, when old-style modesty and marital fidelity are falling out of favor, when nudity and sexual acts of every imaginable kind are presented, verbally and pictorially, in books, magazines, and movies, and when what used to be condemned as "adultery" is widely practiced as "swinging."

How will a couple of such widely differing attitudes ever be able to agree on the upbringing of any children they may have? Perhaps the young wife encourages their little daughter to run about the house and yard naked, while the older husband wants to see the girl "decently dressed." Even if the man's love for his bride helps him to accept all these value differences in her, can he accept her friends, who probably have all her annoying (to him) characteristics and none of her charms? And what will her friends think of him? What will they say about him to her? Here is an anecdote contributed by a friend of mine:

A middle-aged university professor married a secretary twenty years his junior. At the wedding reception, seeking to impress his bride's young friends, he tried to stand on his head in the middle of the floor. He fell and hurt his neck so badly that he had to get medical attention and sleep alone that night. The bride's friends simply laughed at him. The marriage broke up within a few years.

The opposite question arises: Can the young bride accept her husband's friends, people who, because she does not love them, seem to her very old, dull, and prudish? It is a common occurrence for a bride to wean her husband away from the old friends who knew and liked his first wife.

These difficulties are not unusual; they are not unpredictable. Then why do men so willingly risk them? It is because so many men at the climacteric experience the "youth reversion" that I mentioned in Chapter 1. One woman observed it in the husbands of some of her friends: "Their egos soar and they become, or try to become, Don Juans and look for younger women to prove their own youth."

Female Emancipation

Many men still cling to the dogma expressed by Euripides: "A woman should be good for everything in the home, and good for nothing outside it." Some women, of course, agree with Euripides; but increasing numbers of married women disagree and are working outside the home.

Many husbands feel this as a severe threat. It undercuts the man's traditional role as sole breadwinner and so, he fears, weakens his position vis-à-vis his wife and children. It brings the wife into regular contact with other men, which certainly gives her the chance to compare him, perhaps unfavorably, with them. It may, he suspects, give her the temptation, and perhaps the opportunity, to "betray" him sexually. One man reported that, both in his father and in himself, the shock that triggered the onset of the

climacteric symptoms was provided by "independence of wife—
going to work."

Women's roles are changing not only at work but also in bed. It
used to be expected that the bride came to her marriage, if not a
virgin, at least respectably inexperienced in sexual matters. The
groom was supposed to have enough sexual expertise for both
of them and was not required to explain how or where he acquired
it. This was considered normal, natural; the man was assumed to
be more strongly sexed than the woman, equipped by nature to
take the initiative in sexual relationships.

With some couples the woman's reaction to sex—pleasure or
repugnance—was disregarded; those who did consider the
woman's feelings assumed that it was the man's sole responsibility
to see that she was satisfied. Even today, most sex manuals lay
the main responsibility on the man: He is supposed to prolong the
foreplay, to exercise "self-control," and to do whatever else is necessary to ensure the woman's climax. (This is no easy task: For
most men voluntary delay of ejaculation is not under rational control, especially when they are young.)

Such fears were bad enough when a man had to deal only with
his wife. But now, thanks to women's growing sexual freedom,
increasing numbers of men have opportunities to experiment with
erotic relationships. To be sure, this offers the possibility of new
pleasures with new women, but it also presents the risk of failure
and humiliation before these new women. Sexual emancipation for
women, then, leads to increasingly severe strains upon the sexual
capacity of men.

Social Problems

The typical middle-aged man has many relationships outside his
work and his family. He is expected to make certain contributions
to society; he cannot help absorbing certain ideas and behavior
patterns from it. Those relationships may be potent causes of the
climacteric.

Alcohol

It is impossible to know just how many men drink enough alcohol to cause themselves long-lasting physical damage: Many heavy drinkers are secretive about their drinking. But, on such information as I can find, I would estimate that about one million middle-aged men in the United States and about 100,000 in Canada do drink more than is good for them.

There are several reasons. Typically, middle-aged men are more prosperous than young men and can better afford the cost of alcohol. They suffer more social and economic stress than do young men and are likely to move in social and business circles where drinking is an established custom and where the teetotaler is looked on as something of an oddball. Many of them are getting bored with life and find in alcohol an escape from the seemingly dull reality.

So it is that many middle-aged men use alcohol as a tranquilizer for relief from personal, family, and job worries. Some use it as a lubricant to smooth business and social contacts. Others, who might not have any urgent need for alcohol themselves, slip into excessive drinking simply by association with other drinkers, on or off the job.

In many parts of society men are expected to follow the example of Paul the Apostle: "When I was a child, I spake as a child, I understood as a child, I thought as a child: but when I became a man, I put away childish things." This concept of the "child" represents the spontaneous, creative, joyful, playful, hedonistic side of the man's character. The "mature" man puts all that away and by the time he reaches middle age acts a fairly consistent role: "Don't ever be silly." "Watch your dignity." "Don't fool around. No horseplay!" "If you play games, play not for fun but to win." "Men don't pick flowers!" "Men don't show their emotions." "Daddies don't cry!"

But the "child" has not been eliminated—only put away, hidden in the attic. There are times when the child wants out. One time when the "child" can acceptably show itself is when the man is under the influence of alcohol. *Then* his family and friends will not condemn his "silly" behavior; *then* he does not feel ashamed of it: And how enjoyable it is, for a change, to feel young again! This, for many men, is a powerful motive for repeated drinking of alcohol.

I described in Chapter 4 the cause-and-effect relationship between alcoholism and sexual inadequacy. Many men have noticed it in themselves and in their friends. Not so well known is the reverse relationship, in which sexual problems are a cause of excessive drinking. The following are several ways in which men at the climacteric may turn to alcohol.

THE TIMID HUSBAND

J. V. was a master craftsman with a domineering, loud, hard-of-hearing wife. He was psychiatrically described as a "passive-aggressive" personality, which means that normally he was timid and could not stand his ground against the wife, although occasionally, when he had taken a few drinks, they argued and fought.

One thing was good about the marriage: J. V. enjoyed his sex relations with the wife. But when she reached middle age, she lost interest in sex and, in her domineering way, expected him to lose interest, too. J. V. got drunk and found courage enough to force the issue. The wife was furious and, when he sobered up, gave him a severe dressing-down and laid down the law—no more sex, ever! He never dared to defy her again; now he drinks steadily and sleeps alone. Sexual frustration has turned him from an occasional into a habitual drinker.

This pattern is not uncommon. The usually timid, aging husband is repulsed by the dominant, perhaps frigid wife. He drinks more than usual to restore his diminished potency and gain some artificial courage. Feeling ten feet tall and very virile, he asserts his "rights" for what turns out to be the last time. After the showdown, steady drinking and lack of sexual activity soon erode the remains of his virility; he never regains it.

THE BASHFUL LOVER

The bashful lover—perhaps he is unmarried or divorced—suffers from sexual inhibitions; yet from time to time he has managed to get some sexual intercourse. Now, as he reaches middle age, his libido and potency are getting weaker, and the old inhibitions seem stronger. So the next time he is with a woman, he tries a few stiff drinks as an aphrodisiac. He probably fails to achieve intercourse and has a weak erection, loss of erection, or premature ejaculation.

He tries again, with another woman, and with a couple more drinks than before; but of course the more alcohol he consumes, the more his reflexes are dulled and the less potent he becomes. With each failure, he feels more nervous about making another attempt. Shyness—alcohol—sexual inadequacy—increased shyness—more alcohol: It becomes a vicious circle.

This man must choose between sex and the bottle; he can't have both. But whereas sex brings him only embarrassment, the bottle will never laugh at him, will never make him feel inadequate. So he probably chooses the bottle.

THE JEALOUS IMPOTENT

O. B. has been married for some years to an attractive woman, and they have enjoyed a good sex life. Ever since they were courting, he has suffered twinges of jealousy but has eventually come to realize that they were groundless.

Now, with the onset of the climacteric, his libido and potency diminish. He does not understand what is happening to him. Perhaps, with skilled, understanding feminine assistance, he might preserve a fair measure of his sexual powers. But his wife does not know how to help him. Perhaps because of her religion or upbringing, she has always taken a passive role sexually; perhaps they have never talked frankly about sexual matters. Whatever the reason, she says or does nothing now to revitalize their sex life.

Now O. B.'s old jealousy revives; because his wife shows no signs of dissatisfaction, he suspects that she has a lover. He accuses her; she denies it. They quarrel. He goes out and drowns his bitter feelings in alcohol. The scene is repeated again and again. The more fervently she protests her innocence, the more insistently O. B. hammers at his accusations. Believing that his wife has judged him sexually inadequate, he feels utterly humiliated. He takes to drink rather than admit his own sexual inadequacy.

Of course, if he admitted it, he would be able to seek a cure for it. But this is the kind of case that only comes to a doctor much later, for treatment of the damage caused by excessive drinking.

THE GUILT-RIDDEN ADULTERER

D. Y. had been married for twenty years; he was fifty, his wife forty-five, and their daughter sixteen. The marriage had been satisfactory in most ways: He was a good provider, he and his wife shared several common interests and activities, and they had no obvious sexual problems. He was such a light drinker that one bottle of liquor in the house might last as long as two years.

At the age of fifty his behavior began to change. Dinner meetings, formerly three or four a year, gradually increased until they were occurring nearly every week. He came in from these "business meetings" later and later, often quite drunk; and instead of going to bed with his wife, he would sleep on a couch downstairs. He began staying away whole weekends "on business."

Formerly, D. Y. often used to speak lovingly to his wife about herself and about their marriage. Now he began to criticize and sneer: "You don't do anything for me any more. . . . Actually it never was all that hot. . . . There are lots of other women, younger, that would appreciate my looks, and what I have to offer!" She would reply, half-angry, half-joking: "Of course, I can understand how a man would be tempted. I know there are lots of women just waiting for the right man, to have a fling."

Eventually she could no longer close her eyes to what he was up to. He would come home, reeling drunk and bitterly abusive. Next morning he would apologize, but a few days later would repeat the performance. After two years of this, the strain on her was getting unbearable; the daughter was feeling it, too, and was grossly overeating. The wife suggested that they separate, and D. Y. agreed. After living apart for ten months, he asked to come home and promised to quit drinking and abusing her. All went well for a month; then he relapsed.

Now, at fifty-five, he is still living at home, but only to keep his share in the equity of the house and because he finds it physically more comfortable than living alone. He makes no attempt to hide his escapades with younger women. He and his wife never talk about their relationship any more. Even if they could—even if he tried for a reconciliation—it would be too late: She utterly despises him.

A somewhat similar case was that of R. J., as reported by his wife. There was the same beginning: He had a satisfying, seventeen-year-old marriage and two daughters. He was a good husband and father, operated his own successful business, and took only the occasional social drink.

Then at age forty-five came the onset of the climacteric, with a decline in his potency. He began going out, at first occasionally, then more and more often, "to have a drink with the boys." After these sessions he sneaked into the house late at night, and didn't sleep with his wife, because he knew she didn't like his increasingly heavy drinking. At this stage, he really was meeting other men, drinking to drown his anxiety about his waning sexual powers, and nagging and bragging sessions, in which each man tried to cover up the truth about himself but succeeded only in making the others feel worse.

Eventually R. J. met a woman who somewhat restored his faith in his own virility. Now, feeling guilty, he began to treat his wife badly. "He seemed to have changed his entire personality," she said. She was harsh and unforgiving about his drinking and his infidelity. Her criticism drove him to drink even more heavily and eventually to move in with the other woman. The wife tried to cover up for him, pretending to daughters and friends that he was away on business trips.

Before long R. J. became impotent with his mistress, too, and went to his doctor to ask for hormone shots; he got them, but not surprisingly they yielded no results. By that time, his alcoholism had produced cirrhosis of the liver and heart problems; next he developed a bladder tumor that required surgery. His sex life was irremediably ruined.

Eventually R. J. returned to his wife; they established a relationship based on economic expediency—the kind of companionship that is better than loneliness but provides nothing of sex or love.

This pattern, too, can be seen in many men's lives: A good husband and father is unpleasantly surprised by a sharp reduction of potency at the onset of the climacteric. Hoping to regain his virility, he takes to drink and seeks other women. His guilt feelings made him drink more heavily and quarrel with his wife. He rationalizes this by finding imaginary faults in his wife. Unless a reconciliation can be arranged, he continues drinking until his virility, health, and marriage are permanently destroyed.

Here, too, proper advice and treatment when the man first notices his declining virility could avert the whole disastrous sequence of events.

Environmental Stress

Men tend to be exposed more often, and for longer periods of time than women, to environmental stresses, such as excessive noise, strong sunlight, automobile exhaust fumes, and extremes of heat and cold. All such influences produce harmful effects on the body and often on the mind as well. The middle-aged man has less reserve capacity than he did twenty years earlier: His tolerance of all these stresses is less than it was; he feels tired much of the time, and consequently his tolerance for stress is further reduced. For a better-balanced, more healthy life, he should take more time for recreation and rest, but perhaps he cannot or will not do that. So eventually the effects of this stress become unpleasantly noticeable to the man himself and to the people who know him.

Rapid Change

The increasingly rapid rate of change in scientific, technical, and social affairs puts a heavy burden on the middle-aged man. A man's career formerly could be considered as divided into two parts. First came twenty-five to thirty years of hard work and sharp competition; he faced difficulties as a welcome challenge to his abilities. Then, having achieved a good measure of success, he would coast along comfortably, relying on his experience, husbanding his waning strength, basking in the respect of his fellow workers, and enjoying a sense of well-earned security.

Today that simply does not happen in many lines of work. Just when the middle-aged man thinks that he knows the ropes, he finds that the ship is being completely rerigged; most of what he has learned needs updating or complete relearning. Instead of enjoying a secure, prestigious position, he faces a stressful race with younger, more up-to-date competitors who have spent their whole careers in fast-changing conditions and are well adjusted to them.

I heard of a man in his forties who had reached the midmanagement level of a large manufacturing company and then was suddenly challenged because he spoke with a strong foreign accent. "You'll never get any higher in this company while you talk like that!" This unexpected threat to his career seemed to precipitate crises in several aspects of his life: He underwent a major emotional and intellectual upheaval and began attending the "brainwashing" sessions of mystico-psychological organizations. He divorced the mother of his three children (the oldest was nineteen) and married a girl young enough to be his daughter. Then he lived apart from his bride, except for an occasional weekend visit.

The average man finds that by the time he reaches mid-life his powers of adaptation have diminished. He cannot fully adjust as easily as a younger man might, to an age of space-travel, automation, depersonalization, overpopulation, atmospheric pollution, and ecological deterioration.

Increasing Social Involvement

Consider the man in midlife who spends much of his spare time on clubs, professional organizations, community service, politics, and the like. Some of these activities may help to increase his income; through some of them he may feel he is fulfilling his duty as a citizen. Yet all of them take him away from his home, wife, and family, and physical separation often leads to emotional estrangement. The less he sees of them, the less he cares about them.

One man reported that "excitement, like seeing close friends you don't see often, or tense strain, or pressure" would, for him, trigger attacks of physical symptoms of the climacteric, such as poor sexual performance and severe nervous perspiration.

Male Chauvinism

Many men feel the need to brag about their sexual prowess; or if they cannot truthfully brag about it, they will lie about it. They keep this up for two or three decades. The supermasculine frame of mind that demands the bragging and lying will not accept the inevitable, moderate decline of sexuality that accompanies middle age; still less will it accept the severe diminution—in some cases, disappearance—of sexuality that some men experience at the climacteric. There is a widening gap between role and reality, between the imaginary superstud and the actual impotence. It is a severe shock when the man is forced to admit the truth, or perhaps when his wife or girl friend makes some unkind comment about it.

The need to brag, the reluctance to accept the normal aging

process, the shock of newly developed impotence—men have always experienced these things. But there is now another challenge to the traditional myth of male sexual superiority: Today women's sex drives and women's sexual abilities are being more widely discussed. Many men (and women) are surprised to learn that in sexual terms, man is the weaker sex.

Woman is nearly always ready for intercourse, whereas the man must wait until he has an erection. In middle age the erectile center reacts more slowly than it did in youth; so sometimes the man (and the woman) must wait, and wait, and wait for that erection.

If properly stimulated, the woman can have a series of orgasms, one after another. She can remain near the peak of sexual excitement for a long time and repeatedly experience the extra upsurge that brings her to orgasm. On the other hand, the man experiences "resolution," or reduction of sexual excitement, very soon after orgasm and must take a fairly long rest and then go through a whole new cycle of stimulation before he is again ready for intercourse.

See what effect is produced by the dissemination of this knowledge. In the past the standard of sexual accomplishment has generally been set—somewhat like productivity standards in industry—in accordance with the capability of the man involved. That is to say, *the man's* frequency of sexual readiness—perhaps three or four times a week—and *the man's* orgasmic capacity—once and then finished—have been widely accepted as the *right* frequency and the *right* capacity.

What a blow it is to the male ego when a woman says, "No! *My* frequency of readiness—four times a day—is the *right* frequency. *My* orgasmic capacity—many times a night—is the *right* capacity." Is it surprising that a middle-aged man, hearing such heretical theories, may begin to feel insecure and to lose such sexual powers as he had retained?

Fear of Middle Age

In our society many people admire youth as being wonderful in itself. Most of those who have youth flaunt it; many who have lost it try to counterfeit it. Not surprisingly, then, some men fear the approach of middle age. They see the fortieth birthday as the beginning of the end of life. A woman reports, "His fortieth birthday was traumatic for my husband. He disliked the idea of aging, although he had changed very little at that time."

From youngsters, the middle-aged man may hear wounding remarks. "My life's more valuable than yours, Dad; at your age, you're almost dead." From contemporaries he gets frightening folk-medicine tidbits: "You never know about chest pains after you're forty. Have you had an EEG and cholesterol test?" From his own observation he sees that men in their forties are a high-risk group for career dislocations, accidents, extramarital affairs, and divorce.

These influences depress the man and make him increasingly susceptible to many of the physical, mental, and emotional symptoms of the climacteric. Some men try to fool themselves about the passage of time. One man reported "shortness of breath, dimmed eyesight, bulging waistline, smoker's cough, always diagnosed as temporary, never as a sign of creeping aging."

One reason why a man may dread the advancing years is the realization that as he ages, he is becoming a victim of discrimination. He will not, of course, suddenly be barred from voting or from living in certain parts of town; the discrimination is more subtle than that.

Younger people tend to ignore him: They don't talk to him during coffee breaks at work; they don't invite him to their parties. His own children have now left home; they have their own friends, their own interests. If he gets too fond of his grandchildren, he may be accused of spoiling them. He finds that most of the entertainment offered by movies, theaters, night clubs, radio, and television is aimed at people much younger than himself. He sees an abundance of social services—playing fields, clubs, or community centers—aimed at children, young people, or old people and little or nothing intended for him.

Recently it has become acceptable for a middle-aged man to ride a bicycle or run around in shorts. Yet most men would not dare to use a swing or a teeter-totter in the park; they would not dare to roller-skate along the sidewalk. It is small wonder that the middle-aged man sometimes feels nervous and apprehensive, moody, depressed, and irritable; small wonder that he begins to doubt the value of his marriage and his job and so perhaps makes desperate efforts to reshape his life.

Vital Statistics

Considering the facts I have presented in Chapters 5 and 6, one cannot feel surprised that in the United States the average middle-

	United States		Canada	
Cause of Death	45-54 Age Group	55-64 Age Group	45-54 Age Group	55-64 Age Group
Arteriosclerotic and degenerative heart disease				
Male deaths	38,476	77,753	3,341	6,234
Female deaths	9,358	26,634	645	1,884
Stomach ulcer				
Male deaths	425	786	35	67
Female deaths	175	282	9	17
Automobile accidents				
Male deaths	4,144	3,467	410	280
Female deaths	1,675	1,616	181	137
Suicides				
Male deaths	3,007	2,878	263	222
Female deaths	1,405	1,057	106	74
All causes				
Rate per 100,000 males	963.5	2299.7	759.8	1920.3
Rate per 100,000 females	512.2	1105.1	403.3	968.5

aged man must expect to die six years earlier than a woman of the same age. (In Canada, seven years earlier.)

The table on page 132 gives statistics for a few common causes of death. These figures, from the *World Health Statistics Annual,* show numbers of deaths for 1967 and are representative of the state of affairs in recent years.

Such figures indicate a grim state of affairs, from a man's point of view. They are evidence of the increasing level of stress to which men are subjected. In 1920 a man's life expectancy in the United States was only one year less than a woman's. Statistics like these are themselves a source of stress for many of the men who are aware of them; their gloomy message is yet another of the causes that contribute to the climacteric syndrome.

Of course, statistics deal with average men. In the next two chapters I shall offer a number of suggestions that can be used to give an individual man fair prospects of being healthier and living longer than that average.

Part III
PRACTICAL ADVICE

Having described the nature and the causes of the male climacteric, I am now going to suggest what can be done by and for men who are experiencing it. Such men should certainly get competent medical advice, yet they need not leave all the work to the doctor. I shall describe here how climacteric men can cooperate with the doctor for accurate diagnosis and effective treatment.

It is unlikely that a man will experience the climacteric without affecting a number of other people. In Part III I offer those people advice on how to minimize the unpleasant effects and on how to help the climacteric man retain or regain full physical and emotional health.

7

To Men at the Climacteric

After reading Chapters 1 through 6, you may be wondering whether you are at the climacteric. Don't just wonder about it—that can easily lead into worrying and its aftereffects. I am going to suggest a course of action.

First, if you are in the susceptible age group, make a realistic survey of your own physical and emotional condition by filling in the following three charts. Keep in mind what you have read in previous chapters about the various symptoms. Note that I said a *realistic* survey. Don't fall victim to the medical student's disease (*morbus clinicus*) and experience nearly all the symptoms you've read about.

If possible, ask your wife, family, friends and fellow workers whether they have noticed any changes in your health or behavior. Their answers can help you to maintain that realistic attitude; they may also tell you of certain changes that had escaped your attention.

Don't play the hypochondriac and make your own diagnosis. The presence of one or more symptoms from the charts does not necessarily prove that you are experiencing the climacteric. Men do exhibit such symptoms from time to time as part of some illness or condition that has nothing to do with the climacteric. So for a first step just complete the charts. As soon as you get the matter out of your mind and down on paper, it seems less mysterious and frightening.

Symptoms

Column 1 of Chart A gives a list of the sexual, physical, and psychological symptoms described in Chapter 1. Check which of them you experience. In column 2 indicate how long you have been aware of each symptom. In column 3 indicate severity on a scale of 0 to 5, as follows:

0—absent
1—very mild, barely noticeable
2—easily noticeable, causes no real distress
3—sometimes causes distress
4—most of the time causes distress
5—always causes distress

In column 4 if the symptom remains the same or is getting better, reply "No"; if it is getting worse, reply "Yes." In column 5 if any symptom is cyclical, indicate the time between recurrences in days. In column 6 for recurrent symptoms, indicate how long they last on the average on each recurrence, in days.

Chart A: Symptoms

Symptom	How long	Severity	Getting worse	Cycle	Duration
Rarity of erection					
Premature loss of erection					
Premature ejaculation					
Never get erection					
Loss of libido					
Changed sex life					
Urinary irregularities					
Fluid retention					
Hot flashes					
Heart symptoms					

Symptom	How long	Severity	Getting worse	Cycle	Duration
Pseudoangina					
Peptic ulcers					
Itching					
Formication					
Air hunger					
Liver spots					
Headaches					
Backaches*					
Irritability					
Fatigue					
Insomnia					
Moodiness, depression					
Mental difficulties					
Lost self-confidence					
Behavior changes					
Self-delusion					

* I have not named osteoporosis on this chart but have inserted backache, which may be a symptom of that condition and of trouble with intervertebral disks.

PHYSICAL CONDITIONS

Column 1 of Chart B provides a list of the conditions mentioned in Chapter 4. See which of them apply to you. Some of them you may have observed yourself; some may have been diagnosed by your doctor. In column 2 indicate how long you have been aware of each condition. Compute for column 3 on the same scale of 0 to 5 that you used for Chart A:

0—absent
1—very mild, barely noticeable
2—easily noticeable, causes no real distress

3—sometimes causes noticeable distress
4—most of the time causes distress
5—always causes distress

In column 4 if the condition remains the same, reply "No"; if it is getting worse, reply "Yes."

CHART B: PHYSICAL CONDITIONS

Condition	How long	Severity	Getting worse
Hormone decline			
Muscular deterioration			
Arterial deterioration			
Lung deterioration			
Joint and ligament deterioration			
Aging nervous system			
Prostate enlargement			
Eye changes			
Skin deterioration			
Hair graying or loss			
Teeth loss			
Fat accumulation			
Drug or alcohol abuse			

POSSIBLE CAUSES

Some of the symptoms and conditions listed in Charts A and B could perhaps be the results of previous illnesses. If you know or suspect that this is so, enter such under Illnesses in column 1 of Chart C. Then review Chapters 4, 5, and 6 and see which physical, psychological, or social causes may be operative in your life, and enter each one in the appropriate section in column 1.

The following are some causes that one commonly finds operative in middle-aged men. It would be worthwhile to review your own medical history to see if you are or have been subject to any of them:

1. Thyroid or other gland diseases: diabetes, pituitary gland tumor or disease, testicle tumor or disease (perhaps due to mumps), kidney tumor affecting the adrenal glands, thyroid malfunction.

2. Neurological or primary muscle diseases: dystrophy, multiple sclerosis, spinal meningitis, tumors.

3. Rheumatic heart disease; inborn blood vessel abnormalities or injuries (aneurisms, fistulae, shunts)

4. Respiratory problems: emphysema, repeated pneumonia, chronic bronchitis, excessive smoking, pleurisy, injuries, silicosis.

5. Rheumatoid arthritis; injuries or vocational handicaps caused by such jobs as pneumatic drill operating, professional sports, acrobatics.

6. Nerve and brain atrophies; pernicious anemia

7. Cancer of prostate

8. Glaucoma; eye diseases or injuries; eye infections; aneurisms

9. Skin diseases: eczema; allergies; inflammations; irritations; excessive sun exposure; skin cancer

10. Hereditary diseases; deformities or weaknesses

11. Nutritional deficiencies

12. Harmful habituation or addiction: excessive food, drug, or alcohol intake

In column 2 put the date at which the cause occurred or began. In column 3 if the illness or stress continued for a considerable time, indicate how long it lasted.

CHART C: CAUSES

Causes	Date	Duration
Illnesses		
Physical causes		
Psychological causes		
Social causes		

DEALING WITH THE DOCTOR

If the survey you have made on Charts A, B, and C suggests that you may be experiencing the climacteric, make an early appointment with your doctor. Perhaps you have been taking annual medical checkups and are thinking, "If anything was really wrong, my doctor would have noticed it." Maybe so, but he may have missed it: A doctor is not a mind reader or a wizard.

Many ailments are overlooked in medical examinations. Perhaps the patient does not give the doctor all the information about his symptoms. Perhaps the patient forgets some of the details. In some cases the patient is embarrassed to tell the truth: He holds back some of the facts or lies in answer to the doctor's questions about such things as what he eats, how much he drinks or smokes, his sex life, and so on.

The point is obvious: *Tell the doctor everything; don't be embarrassed.* When you see the doctor, give him a copy of Charts A and B, showing the various indications that a change is taking place in your body and your personal life. Does your doctor know about all the items in Chart C? If you are an old patient of his, he probably has those facts on his records; if not, you should mention them. The doctor will probably ask you some questions: Answer them honestly. He is interested not in criticizing or condemning you but in helping you toward recovery.

You may find that your doctor does not accept the existence of a male climacteric at all: Some don't. Some textbooks and specialists use the term but restrict it exclusively to the 15 percent of cases that show a hormonal deficiency. Others, like me, give it a wider meaning.

Don't worry: It does not matter what label is put on your condition. Just ask the doctor to treat your symptoms and advise you how to maintain the best possible general level of health for your age.

Nonhormonal Treatment

Of course I cannot guess what sort of treatment might be required in any individual case, but I will briefly describe the principles and some of the methods that I use. I suspect that many other doctors would proceed in much the same way.

In 85 percent of male climacteric cases there is no hormonal deficiency. Even in the other 15 percent there will probably be some symptoms that are not caused by hormone deficiency. So I would normally apply various nonhormonal treatments first.

The first step is a complete physical examination, with particular attention to the prostate gland. Depending on what this examination reveals, appropriate treatment can be commenced. One man's prostate gland might need special care by a urologist in order to correct urinary or sexual difficulties. Examination will show whether or when an operation is necessary for prostate enlargement. Not every case of enlarged prostate will require surgery, but if an operation is needed, there is no point in postponing it. The most common prostate operation is not normally considered a serious one. It does not, as some people suppose, destroy the man's control over his urination, nor does it leave him impotent or sterile. (There is, however, one type of radical operation that can influence potency.)

Another man's heart and circulatory system will need treatment to restore it to efficient operation; that will probably include a low-cholesterol, low-starch diet and an exercise program. It may also require medication to reduce blood pressure, swelling, chest pain, and shortness of breath. Here, of course, the medication will produce much less than optimum results if the man does not follow the diet and exercise program.

Bone, joint, and disk problems that make a man's movements slow and stiff can be treated by medication, physiotherapy, and postural exercises.

Defective teeth should be cared for. When that is done, the man will look better, will be able to chew his food properly, and hence will digest it better. Improved appearance and improved digestion will contribute towards his feeling better.

For peptic ulcer a medical examination and X ray are essential to discover whether it is caused by excessive tension, by faulty nutrition, or by both. The doctor will advise what should be done to treat it.

As for graying or falling hair, I can suggest no medical remedy. Hair-transplanting operations have succeeded with some men, but they are very costly. Some men find hair dyes and wigs satisfactory, and there is less prejudice now against their use. Yet I think that most men, if they regained full virility and knew they were healthy in other respects, would not worry much about their hair.

Hormone Tests and Treatment

If nonhormonal treatment does not give complete relief, the doctor may suspect premature aging of the testicles, with its accompanying deficiency of male hormones (androgens). There are several methods of testing for this condition.

In tissue sampling of the testicles, a tiny core is taken from one testicle with a hollow needle and examined to see how much or how little testosterone it is producing. This gives accurate results but is rather unpleasant. In my opinion other methods are preferable.

The level of testosterone in the blood can be measured by laboratory testing of a sample. A low testosterone level indicates that the testicles are not functioning adequately.

The level of gonadotrophins in the urine can be measured. Because the output of these hormones may vary widely at different times of day, this test requires collection of all the urine you pass during a twenty-four-hour period. (Obviously that is inconvenient for many men.) As I said in Chapter 4, the gonadotrophins are responsible for stimulating the sex glands. If the level of gonadotrophins is unusually high, the testicles are not responding properly.

Therefore the pituitary keeps increasing its output of gonadotrophins in an attempt to elicit a response.

Unfortunately, very few laboratories are equipped to do tests for testosterone or gonadotrophin levels routinely, and even if you can get them done, they are very expensive. There is a cheaper and faster way that some doctors use. In cases of true hormone deficiency, treatment with testosterone gives quick results: Within a few days the man experiences a reduction of unpleasant symptoms and a dramatic restoration of libido and potency. But testosterone treatment will produce the same results, by a placebo effect, in many men who do *not* have a hormone deficiency. Thus, if the testosterone treatment is correcting a real deficiency, the good results will last for several weeks and can be repeated. If it is only serving as a placebo, the good results will wear off, usually in a few days.

If by one test or another it is determined that you have no hormone deficiency after all, then medical treatment, counseling, and if necessary psychiatric treatment should be sought. If you do have a hormone deficiency, the following discussion outlines how it may be treated.

At first testosterone is usually administered by injection; later on it can usually be given in the form of tablets to be dissolved slowly in the mouth, where they are absorbed by the mucous membrane. (They have little effect if you swallow them.) But taking testosterone alone is usually not advisable. You will remember that in Chapter 4 I described the "thermostat effect," by which, when enough testosterone has been produced, the testicles are temporarily "switched off." We don't want that to happen for the hormone-deficient man: His testicles are not entirely out of action; they are just rather inefficient or "lazy." What we are aiming at is to stimulate those lazy testicles to work as well as they can and then to give just as much additional testosterone as is needed to keep the man at a comfortable level of virility.

The most convenient way of stimulating the testicles is to administer a little of the female hormone estrogen. So if your doctor prescribes estrogen before or along with the testosterone, there's no need to fear that it will feminize you: It is actually an important element of the treatment to preserve and increase your masculinity!

There is one possible danger of hormone treatment: It may speed the development of cancer of the prostate *if you already have it*. Prostate cancer can, in some cases, lie dormant for years or develop so slowly that the patient dies of something else before the cancer gives him any trouble. But testosterone treatment can stimulate one of these dormant cancers into rapid, dangerous growth.

Some doctors view this risk so seriously that they will not use testosterone therapy at all. In my opinion that is being overly cautious: With proper precautions the hormone treatment I have described here is safe and highly effective. But because of the possible risk and because there is in some places a black market in hormones, I offer this warning: *Never take testosterone in any form except when it is prescribed by your doctor.*

I should clarify one more point here. Many middle-aged men, as I mentioned earlier, experience a simple, noncancerous enlargement of the prostate (benign hypertrophy). This affects different cells than does cancer. It rarely turns cancerous, and the existence of this benign hypertrophy is *not* a bar to treatment with testosterone.

Counseling

Many physicians, perhaps through lack of time, had little personal sex experience as students. Few medical schools teach counseling for sexual problems. Sex is studied as a means of reproduction, not as a potential source of happiness or unhappiness. In practice, because of the reticence of patients, and perhaps because of their own reticence as well, physicians do not deal with sex problems as often as would be desirable. Some physicians believe in one or more of the sex taboos described in Chapter 6, and some, deeply involved in their own marital problems, are in no position to give unbiased advice to patients. Even some psychiatrists, gynecologists, and urologists may have little or no training in human sexuality.

But a well-qualified, capable counselor can be very helpful. That's because, in the male climacteric, there is rarely a complete separation of physical and emotional causes. As Shakespeare said:

> We are not ourselves when nature, being oppressed,
> Commands the mind to suffer with the body.

Physical symptoms such as headaches and backaches sometimes accompany depression, for example, and may disappear as soon as the depression is cured. So in most cases counseling or psychotherapy is every bit as effective as medication or other physical treatment.

A sympathetic physician can talk with husband and wife separately, then in joint sessions, to discover and solve marriage problems that may be causing psychosomatic symptoms. He can explain the various changes that they are undergoing, or may expect to undergo, in middle age; he can begin to prepare them for a healthy, happy old age. The doctor may prescribe mood-changing drugs to overcome severe emotional symptoms while he is working to discover and resolve the basic conflicts.

I would emphasize that in these counseling sessions, as in the medical part of your treatment, you should be frank with your doctor: For the best use of your time and his, tell him exactly what you have been feeling and thinking; answer his questions truthfully and fully. Only with such comprehensive information can he decide how best to help you.

What the Doctor Ordered

Many ailments, even after they are correctly diagnosed, linger on needlessly or get worse *because the patient does not follow the doctor's advice* with regard to taking medicine or change of eating, drinking, smoking habits and so on.

To be sure, the reason why some patients don't cooperate is because they don't understand what the doctor is telling them and are ashamed to say so. But it's your business to understand; your health, perhaps your life, may be at stake. If you simply say, "Yes, doctor," and go away, the doctor is entitled to assume that you did understand. So, if you don't understand, ask; and when you do understand, cooperate.

DEALING WITH THE PSYCHIATRIST

If your physician advises you to consult a psychiatrist, here are some hints for making the business as trouble-free and effective as possible.

Many people who go to psychiatrists waste time and money and don't get the best results. The reasons are much the same as those that hamper the physician-patient relationship: The patient, through forgetfulness or embarrassment, does not give all the information he should; or he does not cooperate in carrying through with counseling sessions or interviews. Many men will not involve their sex partners in these sessions.

For example, Jim V. said, "My wife would scream if she knew I was talking to you about our intimate sex life! I could never get her to cooperate: I'd rather put up with things as they are. I could never tell her how I really feel about her: I'd be scared!" Al G. would not dream of cooperating with his wife's psychiatrist because he claimed that "these problems are no outsider's business." He scared his wife so that she would never dare to see her psychiatrist again or even attempt to mention any personal problems to her husband.

For the first interview it would be useful to take along copies of the same three charts you gave to your doctor. A psychological test is often helpful; but it is not always necessary, so if the psychologist does not propose such a test, don't nag him for it. Psychoanalysis is rarely required.

Different psychologists may have different answers to the question, "Is there a true male climacteric?" Some will speak of "a time for self-appraisal in prospective and retrospective terms." Some see it as "a midlife identity crisis." Others prefer the term "involutional depression." It does not really matter what label is applied to your condition: the important thing is that the psychiatrist can help you to recovery from whatever has been bothering you.

He will probably encourage you to discover, and ventilate, whatever emotional conflicts or problems you may have. He may want joint sessions with you and your wife, and perhaps some discussions with her separately. In some cases he may prescribe drugs, such as tranquilizers to suppress anxiety or antidepressants to make you feel more cheerful, perhaps combined with sleeping pills to give you a good night's rest. In some cases of severe depression, shock therapy may be recommended. (Some people have the idea that this is a frightening treatment. In fact, the patient experiences no "shock" at all; he is unconscious, under anesthesia, while an electric current produces a reaction in his brain.)

The psychiatrist-patient relationship is a sensitive one, in which severe personality clashes may develop. If this should happen, the best thing is to switch to another psychiatrist, one with whom you can develop a congenial, helpful relationship. (For some people, a nonpsychiatrist marriage counselor might be preferable.)

Help Yourself

Now I am going to suggest some things you can do to reduce as far as possible the unpleasant effects of the climacteric; they will help you recover from it and go on to a healthier, happier life. You can follow these suggestions in addition to any course of treatment or medication recommended by your own physician, *except* in any instance where one of them obviously clashes with his specific recommendation.

For example, if he says, "Your heart is weak: restrict your physical activity in such-and-such ways," then you will accept that advice and ignore my general encouragement on exercise. Or if your doctor says, "You must not eat this, that, and the other," then you will plan your diet accordingly, instead of following my suggestions about food.

If you are approaching the susceptible age but have not yet felt any climacteric symptoms, you too would do well to follow these suggestions. Thus you may delay the onset of the climacteric, make it much milder when it does come, or with luck avoid it altogether.

Diet

For a middle-aged man, the two aims of a correct diet must be to bring his weight to the optimum level for his height and build and hold it there and to ensure that his entire body is soundly nourished.

There is no need for me to give specific instructions: plenty of excellent material on diet is available in other books and in pamphlets distributed by public-health authorities. For advice on how to choose among all this material, ask your doctor—and beware of unscientific fad diets.

It is sometimes difficult to make major changes in one's diet when cultural influences or long-established habits are involved, and especially when family tastes or social obligations interfere. The best way is to get the whole family menu adjusted so that, with suitable variations in quantity, all members can share the same meals rather than going to the trouble of preparing two or three different diets. Get your wife to keep forbidden food items right out of the kitchen; then you will not be tempted to eat what you shouldn't.

Exercise

In Chapter 4 I mentioned loss of muscle tone as a major influence in general physical (and sexual) degeneration. That loss can be prevented or lost muscle tone can be restored by regular exercise. (But watch your disks and your heart.) Here too plenty of good, informative books and pamphlets are available; your doctor will advise you.

Many middle-aged men have found it helpful and enjoyable to join a club or other organization where, under trained supervision, they can pursue a regular exercise program in company with other men of their own age group.

Work

I described in Chapter 6 several ways in which excessive work can contribute to the onset and continuation of the climacteric. Here is a program of action that will markedly reduce or even eliminate this harmful influence.

If your job is hopelessly uncongenial, get another. One can hardly overestimate the emotional and physical harm caused by spending half your waking hours under the stress of fear, boredom, resentment, or whatever unpleasant reactions you suffer from a job you hate.

Lost seniority or pension rights, the problems of finding, learning, or getting used to the new job, even a reduction of income—none of these is too high a price to pay for the benefits you will gain.

I remember the case of a high school teacher in his forties who was bored and dissatisfied with his work. He resigned from the school and went to work, eight hours a day, in a metal smelting plant. Although the work is physically harder, he finds it emotionally less tiresome: He has more mental energy to enjoy his hobbies. He has enough spare time to be a scoutmaster. In some people's eyes, perhaps, the man's new job carries less prestige, but he finds his life happier and healthier than it was.

Perhaps you enjoy your work but have become excessively involved with it, to the point where you are sacrificing rest, recreation, and family. Then cut down on the time, thought and energy you give to your work; give more to the nonworking aspects of life. To cut down work volume and responsibility and to shorten working hours are particularly important for peptic ulcer patients. (For most self-employed men it's an excellent idea to do it without waiting to develop peptic ulcers or other psychosomatic ailments.)

It's worth a reduction of income, if necessary, to restore a better balance to your life. Aim to divide your day into eight hours of work, eight hours of recreation (including meditation), and eight hours sleep. Your friends and your wife will appreciate the chance to see more of you; the greater personal freedom, the added time available for recreation and for your family, are powerful healing factors.

A woman reported, concerning her husband, "Shortly after his fortieth birthday he was denied a promotion that he felt he had earned, and no explanation was given. We all felt it was unfair. Later (about three years) he accepted the situation and rather enjoys the diminished responsibility and added free time." For employees it is wise to consider carefully the pros and cons of any promotion that is offered. If on analyzing the new position you find that it would be overdemanding, refuse it! The decision may be difficult at the time, but in the long run it may save your health.

Put these questions to yourself when you are considering this matter of excessive absorption in work:

How many meals do you eat with your family each week?
How many evenings do you spend together each week?
Do you have ample time for holidays with your family?
Where do you spend most of your time?
Do you fear a change because you think society is prejudiced against age and may refuse you a new job?

If you are afraid of retirement, there's a simple way to conquer the fear: Begin to *plan* for retirement. Begin to train yourself for a new career, if that's what you fancy. If not, begin to plan, save, and study if necessary for whatever leisure-time activities you intend to pursue.

Leisure

Are you fully satisfied with the way you use your leisure time? I should emphasize that leisure, to my mind, is not just laziness or inaction: It is the time when you really do your "living"; it yields true re-creation, in the sense of making yourself anew. If you are not satisfied, compile a list of five things you would like to do with your leisure and make specific plans for achieving them.

Here is a striking example of the therapeutic effect of leisure. A middle-aged man came to me complaining that he had become nearly impotent. "Actually, my wife doesn't like sex," he said, "and she's glad about what's happened to me. But *I'm* not glad, and I want something done about it!" Examination indicated no specific ailments. The man wanted hormone shots, so we tried them with no success. The man stayed upset, the wife stayed happy.

The man was self-employed and had not taken a vacation for years. I persuaded him to get away from his business for three weeks. He and his wife went to Hawaii. On his return he reported, "Doctor, the second day we were there, I got my sex drive and virility back again, to the point where I had to have intercourse every night."

The wife, although she could not share his sexual enthusiasm, was happy for him. The improvement did not continue after his return to work; but at least the man now understands the cause of his problem and is going to make sure that from now on he gets regular vacations.

Emotional Habits

I have mentioned such things as irritability, moodiness, depression, and self-doubt as symptoms of the climacteric. These are, in most cases, only habits, habits that were formed by repetition of certain negative thoughts and feelings. Such habits can be broken and replaced by constructive, enjoyable habits of thought and feeling that will keep you, most of the time, calm, cheerful and self-confident. The new good habits are formed, like the bad old ones, by repetition.

Suppose, for example, that you have been bothered by oft-repeated thoughts and fears of aging, sickness, and death and are now going to replace them with something positive and constructive. You can make up your mind to accept your present age as a good one. Think back on various bygone problems; let yourself feel thankful that you have now overcome them. Dwell on the various benefits of your present time of life and let yourself feel pleased with them. Think forward to some good, enjoyable things that you expect to do in the near future; if there aren't any, then get busy and plan some.

Another example is the many men who are apathetic all the time—they never feel enthusiastic about life, people, work, pleasure, or anything at all. Yet they can cultivate enthusiasm. Enthusiasm is not a quality that some people possess innately while others lack it. There is a spirit in every man that is capable of generating enthusiasm for life and living. Try to look at life with a new attitude; let go of doubts and fears about yourself, your life, and your affairs; open yourself to positive, constructive ideas. Think back to occasions in the past when you did feel enthusiasm; remember what it felt like and deliberately try to re-create the same feeling.

With a well-directed effort, you can become enthusiastic about your work, about the people you meet, about all the opportunities to give, to learn, and to develop that are constantly being presented to you. Prosperity is a process of growth and fulfillment; it is all around you, but you must claim it.

When you have improved your attitude toward life, you will find it not too hard to change your thinking about age and death. It is possible to look forward to retirement rather than dread it; you can accept death as part of life, not the end of it.

Constructive change in your habits of thought and emotion will be eased and speeded if you take some kind of action that will help the process. For example, if you want to develop self-confi-

dence, take a course in public speaking. Many middle-aged men
have found religion a powerful therapeutic influence: You could
perhaps return to a religious faith you had abandoned, or you
could try investigating a number of religions until you find one that
meets your needs.

A change of emotional habits is often essential for successful
treatment of climacteric symptoms (and for other conditions, too).
Consider, for example, three stages of digestive disorder: "nervous
stomach," hyperacid gastritis (excessively acid stomach, with
inflammation), and peptic ulcer (of esophagus, stomach, or duodenum). A physician would probably prescribe tranquilizers, with
or without spasmolytics (drugs to suppress stomach spasms) and
antacids (chemicals to reduce or neutralize stomach acid), and an
ulcer diet.

Yet the most important feature of the treatment must be supplied by the patient himself (perhaps with the aid of psychotherapy): He must recognize and change the attitudes and situations
that are producing stress in his life. This may require the adoption
of new moral, social, and economic values; it may require the
discarding of perfectionist or excessively competitive work methods; it may even necessitate a change of job or a move to an
entirely new environment.

Premature Ejaculation

Premature ejaculation is not normally produced by physical
causes but by deep-seated psychoneurotic influences that would
need psychiatric exploration and treatment. Nevertheless, I will
offer some encouraging thoughts. This is a problem that tends to
decrease as you grow older. With advancing age, the ejaculation
naturally becomes less violent and more prolonged. One corre-
spondent wrote, "the sex act . . . is changing: The feeling or form
of orgasm is now (while very beautiful at the best occasions) not
as explosive. It is rather suffused over a little more time, less
thrusting out, more inundating. Hard to describe!"

Another change is that many older men are able to rise to a high level of sexual excitement and yet retain enough self-control to refrain from ejaculating. This enables them to prolong the sex act and so give greater satisfaction to their partners.

PROSPECTS FOR THE IMPOTENT MAN

I discussed in Chapters 4 and 5 the two types of impotence: physical impotence, produced in about 2 percent of cases by surgery or physical injury; and psychological impotence, about 98 percent of cases. Let's look at the prospects for men with these two conditions.

Physical Impotence

First let me assure the man who has lost the physical ability to get an erection that *his sex life is not over*. His hormonal output and brain functions remain normal; so he is no less virile, no less passionate than he was before the injury or surgery. He can adapt old methods of sexual expression, and if necessary learn new ones, to satisfy his wife or lover and to fulfill his own sexual needs.

A major handicap for many men is that they have come to accept a narrow definition of sexual intercourse as consisting of the penetration of the vagina by the penis. Indeed, this is just about all that many couples achieve; yet it is only a part, and for most women the least important part, of the full process of intercourse.

Many women prefer stimulation of the clitoris, labia, and vagina by manual or oral caresses to ordinary coitus. There are many men, too, for whom coitus is less enjoyable than having the woman stimulate their erogenous zones and sexual organs with her hands, lips, and tongue.

I was not too surprised to read in the periodical *Medical Aspects of Human Sexuality* reports of an investigation showing that oral stimulation was practiced by about 50 percent of the couples interviewed, at least as a part of their sexual foreplay.

Why is this not more widely known and more widely discussed among men? Somehow the conventional concept of masculinity has become centered upon coitus; for some reason these other forms of sexual activity are considered by many men sissified, dirty, or taboo.

The middle-aged man with physical impotence would do well to drop any such inhibitions. He and his wife ought to explore all possible varieties of love play, perhaps reviving techniques they have not used for years or if necessary learning and perfecting techniques that they have never tried before. In this way they have excellent prospects of revitalizing the sexual aspect of their relationship.

Psychological Impotence

Take heart from this fact: Of the 98 percent of potency problems that are psychological in origin, most can be treated. Get a complete physical checkup and proceed to correct all health problems that are discovered. Your physician may also recommend marriage or family counseling. I offer below a number of ideas that you can consider and apply as long as they do not clash with any specific advice you have received from physician or counselor.

First, you may have to revise your concept of the male-female sex relationship. You may have some false notions—perhaps left over from boyhood days—about female sexuality and the woman's role in love and marriage. For example, some men still think that the woman's duty is simply to submit to the man's sexual advances whenever he feels like using her. She has no right to demand pleasure for herself from sex; she herself should not initiate any sexual activity.

This is wrong. Sexual intercourse is a pleasure that should be mutually desired and mutually enjoyed. Either partner should feel free to ask for it by word, look, or action; either should feel free to refuse it, for personal reasons, without fear of resentment by the other.

Second, you may have to revise your concept of what is sexual intercourse. As I said above, intercourse is *not* simply the insertion of penis into vagina to the accompaniment of a few gasps, groans, and convulsive movements. Intercourse, in the full meaning of the term, is a whole galaxy of actions that the couple engage in for mutual erotic fulfillment.

The foreplay leading up to the actual sexual climax should ideally include most of the hours of the day that the couple spends together. Wooing, or courtship, might sound rather old-fashioned to some men, something that they did years ago, before they were married, and promptly abandoned when married.

Third, you may have to get rid of some false ideas that you have a sex quota to fulfill—a certain number of sex acts per week. This is a false approach. You do *not* have to compare yourself with yourself in young manhood or with reports (probably inflated) of what other men achieve in bed.

The mature middle-aged man will not try to outdo a twenty-year-old in the sexual sphere any more than he would try it on the track or in the swimming pool. The important questions for the middle-aged man are: "Am I satisfying my own sexual needs?" and "Am I satisfying the sexual needs of my wife?"

For satisfaction, quality is more important than quantity. Once you stop trying to keep numerical tally, you can become more interested in a refined sex life that is sensually and esthetically satisfying to both partners. This is like the connoisseur who gets more pleasure from a few drinks of good wine than he would from swilling pints of rotgut.

I know I said earlier that a woman's sexual capacity is theoretically greater than a man's. Nevertheless, most women do show some decline in sexual capacity as they advance in years: They cannot resume their cycle of response so quickly as they did twenty-five years earlier. Indeed, by middle age, the two sexes are more nearly compatible, sexually, than they were in their twenties: They both need more time to prepare for a repetition of the sex act.

This is an excellent reason, by the way, for a man over forty to avoid marrying a woman young enough to be his daughter and to choose one closer to his own age. He might even consider reestablishing his sexual confidence and with his wife relearning and rediscovering the arts of courtship and lovemaking.

Fourth, a powerful stimulus to sexual excitement is to bring up and dwell fondly upon the memories of previous enjoyable sexual experiences. Men may often get erections at inconvenient times by doing this, but it's a technique that can be developed for use whenever you need it.

Once the pattern of sexual arousal and behavior has been established in those parts of the brain and nervous system that control the erection center, it remains fixed there; on an appropriate stimulus, it will go into action again and again. The more often you apply this stimulus, the quicker, stronger, and more reliable will be the response; in this, as in many other physical and mental acts, practice makes perfect.

Fifth, in Chapter 5 I emphasized the deadening effect of monotony on a couple's sex life. The obvious remedy for this is to bring *variety* into your sex life. Variety of sexual encounter is the first suggestion. Books and marriage counselors can provide ideas; some men would be surprised what ideas their wives could offer if encouraged to speak out. Then there's room for variety of time and place: Break the every-Friday-at-10-o'clock habit. The second honeymoon method has rejuvenated many men.

Sixth, in every aspect of this campaign, bear in mind that the one safe and reliable aphrodisiac is sexual activity. I emphasize that this term "sexual activity" does *not* apply only to coitus: I am using it in the broadest possible sense to include also thinking, hoping, remembering, dreaming, looking, touching, talking, reading books, seeing movies—anything and everything that, for you, has any pleasurable connection with sex. The more gratifying sexual activity you have, the more you enjoy it; and you'll find that the more you enjoy it, the greater becomes your capability.

Seventh, development of free, frank communication between

the man and woman can be a powerful stimulus. To some readers this may sound obvious; yet in fact much sexual difficulty is caused by a lack of mutual understanding. Many couples never communicate well enough to realize that male and female sexual responses are quite different, especially with regard to what each experiences as "sexual satisfaction."

The man should not expect the woman to have the same orgasmic experience as he does; if she does not behave during coitus in the way he expects, he should not assume that he is failing her. The man should learn to accept joyfully whatever pleasure he derives from their sexual relationship; he should allow the woman to do the same without feeling personally responsible for the quality and intensity of her gratification.

Women who have grown up with ideas of equality of the sexes may feel free to take the first steps to establishing this kind of communication. Some middle-aged women did not grow up with these ideas, so I suggest that for many middle-aged couples it is the man's responsibility to speak up and to say and do, tactfully and lovingly, whatever is necessary.

Finally, many men court, marry, and become fathers without any clear idea of what "love" means. (Of course, many women are in the same boat; but at the moment I am addressing the men.) A good provider is not necessarily a good lover. A highly virile, highly potent man is not necessarily a good lover. Love is not just an emotion, like fear, hatred, or anger. Love is not something that comes to you from an external source, like a sunburn, a frostbite, or an attack of measles.

The problem with many middle-aged married men is not that they originally chose the wrong wives (as so many of them believe) but that a formerly satisfactory marriage has been allowed to go sour. How many middle-aged men realize that love is an art—like singing, acting, and painting—an art that requires training and practice in the beginning, plus constant reviewing and upgrading? How many middle-aged men would bother to court their wives now, as they courted them before marriage, to practice and encourage their wives to practice the arts of mutual seduction and mutual enticement? Such practices could revitalize many marriages.

Seventy percent of men who get divorced at the age of forty-five or older are not really tired of women or of marriage: They quickly marry again. If in the second marriage they apply the ideas I have mentioned in the preceding pages, they may hope to find happiness; but if they repeat in the second marriage the same mistakes that spoiled the first, they will experience the same unhappiness that already drove them to the divorce court. For many men it would be better to use the principles mentioned in this chapter to make a sincere effort to salvage the first marriage.

8

Help for the Climacteric Man

This chapter is intended for those people—wives, daughters, sons, friends, fellow workers, employers, and so on—who have to live with or deal with men at the climacteric. It may assist you to understand these men, to help them, and to protect your own interests.

WOMEN

For the woman who loves a man, it is distressing to see him start manifesting the symptoms and behavior changes that I described in Chapter 1. Feeling anxious does no good to you or to him, but there are several helpful things you can do.

Recognize the Climacteric

Many women do not know that men experience the climacteric, and because they don't know about it, they are blind to the signs of it. One woman who had worked for years in the medical field said to Raymond Hull,

> It's very common that men should start looking around at forty, for all sorts of reasons, to prove that they're still male. But I've not seen any organic signs, the way you can in a woman. Men, for example, don't appear to have hot flashes, or any of the

obvious things that go along with hormonal change. I've never thought about it.

Now many men *do* have hot flashes and the obvious signs that go along with hormonal change. But because this woman had never heard any man complaining about such symptoms (as I said earlier, many men are reluctant to mention them), she had never thought about the subject.

Lost potency or lost libido alone do not prove that the man is experiencing the climacteric. He may be generally run down in health. He may be worried about work, money, politics, his children, his parents, or the state of his soul. Any of these causes may, for longer or shorter periods, suppress a man's sexuality.

The man may simply be bored with his sex life. There's a perfectly natural tendency to get bored with anything, including sex, that is repeated often enough with no variation. In many marriages it is the wife who creates and maintains this sex boredom: She will adopt only the one position for intercourse; she will not permit any foreplay; she will not manually stimulate the man; and she will certainly not give him oral stimulation. (I know that many men are equally unenterprising; but I have offered some advice to them elsewhere.)

Remember then, that the dwindling of a man's sex drive does not by itself prove that he has reached the climacteric. But if you notice several of the signs described in Chapter 1—for example, one sexual, two or three physical, and two or three psychological symptoms—you have reasonable cause to suspect that he is experiencing the climacteric.

Discussion

If you have been in the habit of speaking frankly to each other about personal problems, there will be no difficulty now in discussing the state of your husband's health. (An easy way to bring up the subject is to show him this book; suggest that he read it and fill in the self-analysis charts in Chapter 7.) In this analysis and discussion, bear in mind what I said in Chapter 5 about the false concept of dualism, the theory that mind and body are separate entities. The medical profession is gradually accepting the fact that man is not a duality but one whole being.

I have had to describe separately the various causes and symptoms of the climacteric, but they are not really separate and cannot be treated separately. The physical, mental, and emotional are all delicately intertwined; for best results they must be diagnosed and treated together.

If he has been in the habit of getting regular medical checkups, there will not now be much difficulty in getting him to see the doctor. Even if he goes reluctantly, that is better than not going at all.

A man came to me: "I don't know why I'm here. I'm not worried about myself, but my wife thinks there's something wrong, and she wants me to talk to the doctor about it." "What does your wife think is wrong with you?" I asked him. "I've lost all interest in sex. I don't really miss it, but it bothers her; so she thought I ought to do something about it."

It is often helpful if the wife makes the appointment for her husband, goes to the doctor herself in advance, and gives him a description of her husband's condition as she sees it. That precaution will prepare the doctor for the man's visit; it will guard against the possibility that the man may not be frank in describing his symptoms to the doctor. It is also helpful if the man is genuinely unaware of some of his symptoms (for example, personality changes).

Suicide?

Suppose that your observation, whether supplemented or not by discussion with your husband, gives you grounds to believe that he is experiencing the climacteric. I don't want to arouse needless alarm; yet it must be admitted that some men in this condition do become disturbed enough to kill themselves (like Raymond Hull's doctor friend, mentioned in the Introduction). In most countries where statistics are available, suicide rates for men show a sharp rise beginning in the mid-forties. It is not unreasonable to assume that many of these suicides are caused by the stresses of the climacteric.

Before they actually do the deed, most suicides give various clues that indicate their state of mind. If you know what clues to look for, you may well be able to save the man's life.

First, don't swallow the old fallacy: "Those who threaten to kill themselves never do it." This is the exact reverse of the truth: In reality, nearly every suicide talks about it in advance. Even apparently casual remarks about suicide should be taken seriously.

Second, suicides, whether or not successful, are nearly always preceded by mental depression.

Third, the suicide typically has a feeling—it may or may not be justified—of emotional isolation; he has come to believe that nobody cares about him, that nobody minds whether he is healthy or sick, happy or unhappy, alive or dead. Words or acts indicating this isolation may be significant.

Fourth, preparation of the means of death is often a clue: Purchase of firearms and ammunition or the overhauling of a long-neglected gun and the accumulation of lethal quantities of drugs are examples of clues.

Fifth, there are thinly disguised suicide techniques, such as habitual dangerous driving, participation in dangerous sports, and excessive consumption of food, tobacco, or alcohol.

If your observation suggests that a man may be considering suicide, don't delay. Consult your doctor at once, and get his recommendation as to treatment. If you cannot do that, then many cities have suicide prevention clinics that you can phone twenty-four hours a day for advice.

Peptic Ulcers

For a married man the cure of peptic ulcers depends upon three things: timely medical treatment; personal adherence to the prescribed diet, medication, and life-style; and full cooperation by wife and family. The following are some general hints for carrying out the last item.

It is best if the whole family can modify its diet and mealtimes, at least to some degree, to fit in with the man's prescribed menu and schedule. This helps him to feel less like an invalid, makes mealtimes more pleasant for him, and so reduces the stress on his digestive system.

Take all resonable steps to avoid annoyances and irritations in the home. This does not mean repressing all mention of problems: It requires that problems be brought into the open and discussed as calmly and reasonably as possible. Better still, try to eliminate, as far as is practicable, the causes of annoyance. It is worth a radical rearrangement of your living habits to achieve this.

Appropriate physical exercise is helpful in many ulcer cases. For many men this would be more interesting and enjoyable if they could share the exercise with their wives; and the exercise that is enjoyable is likely to be better sustained, and will certainly be more beneficial, than some kind of activity that is done alone, from a grim sense of duty.

For a complete, permanent cure, the man has to make a lasting change in his entire mental attitude. This change is never going to be easy, but it can be made much less difficult if the woman is willing to modify her mental attitude, too. Habits of thought and speech are infectious. The wife can in this way greatly help her husband (and as a bonus she will find her own life becoming more pleasant, too).

B. B. worked for a large mining and smelting company, earning excellent wages. He developed peptic ulcers and in spite of medical treatment showed no improvement, lost weight, and continued to look and feel miserable.

Personal counseling revealed a severe conflict in his life, springing from his bitter dislike of the work he was doing. I said, "So you hate your present job! Then, if you could have your way, what would you like to do?" "My life's dream," he replied, "was to build a boat and sail around the world." "Why don't you do it?" "I feel I have to provide security for my wife and family; so I stick to my job at the smelter." "Have you ever spoken to your wife and family about your ambitions?" "No; I never have. I don't think they would go for it."

I persuaded him to hold a family council and to speak his mind. The wife and children didn't raise the objections that he had feared: It was decided to sell the house, build the boat, and live on it. They now sail for six months of each year and return to Canada for the other six, during which time both parents work and give travel lectures to earn money for the next six-month cruise. B. B.'s ulcers have disappeared, his family is healthy, and they are all happily sharing an exciting life.

Better Than Nothing

The advice I've offered so far in this chapter is based on the assumption that the woman can frankly talk to her husband about his health problems. Unfortunately, in many cases it's not so easy. In Chapter 2 I mentioned two common difficulties: The wife dare not raise the subject of her husband's health, or they do discuss it, but the husband refuses to go to the doctor.

If for these or any other reasons you cannot get your husband to see the doctor, the next-best thing is to go to the doctor yourself. See Charts A, B, and C at the beginning of Chapter 7. Fill them out, as well as you can, with the facts concerning your husband and take them with you. This will make the consultation as useful as possible, and will improve your prospects of getting some helpful advice.

Renewed Sex Life

For many women the most disturbing feature of the male climacteric would be the impairment or termination of a formerly enjoyable sex life caused by the sexual symptoms described in Chapter 1.

Medical or psychiatric treatment can in most cases do much to eliminate the symptoms; but the effect of such treatment can be accelerated and increased through a wife's loving, active cooperation. The following are some suggestions that I would offer to women in this position.

First, many people—probably more women than men—are still influenced by old-fashioned, antihedonistic notions concerning sex. Such theories, depicting sex as a duty not a pleasure, may have had a sound basis at one time, in societies where lifelong, monogamous marriage was the rule and where contraception was unknown.

These notions should be reviewed and as far as possible abandoned. Sex is not merely a biological release of primitive urges; it is not simply a bit of mild therapy, like an enema or a mouthwash, serving to clean out a part of the body once in a while. Sex should be thought of, and experienced, as a means of enriching the whole of one's life, as the ultimate physical and emotional expression of the union of two persons.

Second, there are a lot of traditional prejudices regarding the role of the man as initiator and aggressor in sexual activity. Many women, and men, feel that it is solely the man's responsibility to get sexual pleasure for himself and to provide pleasure, if he can, for the woman. She is supposed to lie passively and enjoy herself or, if she can't enjoy herself, lie there and pretend to enjoy herself while she is really planning tomorrow's shopping list.

These prejudices should be abandoned. For fully satisfying sexual relations, both partners must take an active part. No man loses any of his virility by letting his wife take some or all of the initiative to aid his diminishing sex drive. A woman loses none of her dignity or femininity by taking action to re-create romance that seems to be fading.

Of course, it's best if the woman has been taking an active sexual role before the man enters the climacteric. So don't wait until he begins to exhibit the climacteric symptoms: Start now.

Third, for the purpose of saving the sexual side of a marriage—and this may be decisive in saving the entire marriage—a wife should not hesitate to review her concepts of what is permissible or "normal" in sexual relations.

Many a wife does hesitate. Perhaps the husband buys her some exotic-looking lingerie and asks her to wear it. Perhaps he suggests that she should sometimes act differently—maybe assume a dominant role—in their sexual encounters. Or perhaps he proposes some sort of act that she has thought of as a "perversion." The wife may go on the defensive: "What's wrong? Don't you love me just the way I am?" She may stall. She accepts the lovely nightgown but puts it away "for some special occasion"—an occasion that never comes. Or she proposes delaying the sexual experiments "until your next vacation, when we have more time" and, of course, during his vacation, they still have only the same old twenty-four hours a day. She may turn hostile: "All you ever think about is sex!"

Such a woman urgently needs counseling. She must be helped to understand that there are no "wrong" techniques for sex. Whatever produces mutual pleasure and satisfaction for a couple is "right" for them. She must realize that sex is not something to be restricted to one room and one particular time of day: I have mentioned elsewhere the concept of the "all-day sex act," for which the partners begin to arouse each other hours before they go to bed.

The woman who rejects these ideas, who refuses to cooperate with her husband in obtaining a richer, more satisfying sex life, runs the risk of driving him into the arms, and the bed, of another woman who will do so.

Fourth, it is important that the partners should be able to discuss frankly any influences that might impair their sex life; they should also feel free to put forward proposals for improving it. I know that for some couples this is not easy. One woman summed it up thus:

> I feel it takes patient sensitivity on the part of a woman to understand a man—to know when he needs help and when he wants to be left alone. To be too insistent will make him irritable and reluctant to discuss his sexual symptoms. Yet at times he does need a partner there, to listen to his problems; and at times he appreciates the encouragement of a feminine woman.

This sort of communication can be achieved; it is worth making one's very best efforts to do so, perhaps with the help of a sympathetic physician or therapist.

OTHER RELATIVES

This section is directed to parents (many people today live long enough to see their sons reach the climacteric age), sisters, brothers, sons, daughters—to anyone who has a familiar relationship with the climacteric man. To you I make the same preliminary suggestion that I gave the wives: Be alert for the signs of the climacteric.

Suppose you see the signs. If the man has a wife, it's in most cases best to mention the subject to her first; if he has no wife, then raise the subject directly with him. (For you, as for the wives, giving him a copy of this book might be an easy way to do it.) Use whatever influence you have to persuade him to go to the doctor for examination and treatment.

EMPLOYERS AND FELLOW WORKERS

I described in Chapter 3 some of the difficulties that the climacteric may cause for the man at work; it also creates many difficulties for his employer and fellow workers. My first suggestion is this: If the man shows sudden personality changes or a sudden decline in his ability to do the work, don't assume that he is losing interest in the job. Don't assume that he is just aging: The normal aging process produces only *gradual* changes of personality and ability.

The changing of jobs, although you often see it in men of this age, can guarantee no lasting solution; often the man takes his problems with him to the new job. This situation is parallel to the climacteric man's restless search for new women: There, too, he is merely transferring the old problems to a new environment.

It is far better to find out what is wrong here and now: It may be the climacteric. If you can, talk to the man about it; show him this book. If you have enough influence or authority, get him to see a doctor.

The climacteric need not signal the stagnation or the ruin of a man's career. There are good prospects that, with proper treatment, he can regain his former personality, interests, and abilities and be fit for many more years of productive, satisfying activity.

A. K. was a foreman steamfitter, successful and prosperous: He owned a house, car, boat and camper; he took frequent fishing trips and regular vacations; he enjoyed his work and seemed to have no higher aspirations. He was married twice; his first wife had remarried after the divorce, and his children by her were grown up and independent. He himself had remarried at fifty and had a young son by his second wife. He was energetic and cheerful and seemed to have just about everything a man could want.

At fifty-four his personality began to change: He had spells of fear and restlessness, alternating with depression and apathy. His mental processes deteriorated; he could not concentrate, could not read or watch television, and lost the ability to make decisions (there were mornings when he could not even make up his mind to put on his pants). He began to suffer from sweating spells, dizziness, and buzzing in the ears. At work he became fearful of responsibility and had to step down from his foreman's post to a lower position. At home he became afraid to entertain friends. He completely lost his sex drive. He sat alone, brooding on the futility of life and the approaching end, the downhill slope to the grave.

The family doctor tried unsuccessfully to counsel and medicate him. He was referred, in turn, to three psychiatrists. The first declared that he could find no psychopathology. The second psychiatrist said that A. K. liked to be miserable, that he was deriving "secondary benefits" from being pampered and mothered by his wife, and that he did not really want to get better. The third psychiatrist could not understand why A. K. was depressed but gave him a number of shock treatments and prescribed antidepressant drugs; the drugs did blot out some of A. K.'s troubles, but they also made him forget a number of other things worthy of being remembered.

None of these psychiatrists ever discussed with A. K. the question of his lost identity or the apparent purposelessness of his life. At last the family doctor realized that the case was being mismanaged and began a new treatment of weekly hormone injections and group therapy.

After four hormone shots, the unpleasant physical symptoms— the sweating, buzzing, dizziness, and so on—were cleared up; by the fifth week his sexual potency was fully restored. The group sessions gave new meaning and dimensions to his life and helped him to build a new identity even more satisfying to himself and his family than was his former self.

Voters and Politicians

It is not safe to assume that the man appointed or elected to public office at forty will remain through several decades the same in character and capability. The male climacteric may at any time undermine his ability to withstand the physical stresses of his post; it may upset his mental and emotional equilibrium to the point at which he cannot do the work he is supposed to do.

A judge who has to keep adjourning court so that he can urinate, a legislator who cannot concentrate on the debate because of his chronic itching, a labor arbitrator who is thinking more about his own incessant headache than about the rights and wrongs of the dispute before him, a diplomat whose former suavity has turned into chronic irritability, a head of state whose former confident, decisive character has altered to one of timidity and procrastination—these are all a few examples of the possible effects of the climacteric.

Voters and colleagues in office should be on guard. The stakes are high—not just the happiness of one wife and a couple of children, but in some possible cases the fate of a nation. Voters and colleagues will not normally have access to the medical records of the men involved. Voters may rarely, or never, even have the chance to see the man in person. But there are three signs that are significant.

The first sign is noticeable personality change, in which the man suddenly begins to show some of the mental and emotional symptoms described in Chapter 1. The signs might be sudden, drastic changes of clothing, grooming, or general life style.

The second sign is a sudden, noticeable decline in the ability to transact public business or to carry out whatever may be the duties of his office. This may be the outward manifestation of physical, mental, and emotional symptoms that otherwise could not be detected by outsiders.

Third, a sudden upset of a formerly stable personal life is another indication. This might be shown by such signs as the breakup of a long-established and apparently happy marriage or a sudden religious conversion.

It is customary that for many important posts the candidate will undergo a medical examination. Yet the examination may in reality only determine whether or not the man is in any serious risk of an early death. It may not, unless special attention is directed to that point, indicate whether or not the candidate is suffering from the climacteric. Climacteric symptoms are particularly likely to be overlooked if they are intermittent or cyclical. Moreover, even if a full examination shows that the man is not now experiencing the climacteric, that is no guarantee that he will not begin to experience it next month or next year.

I would not presume to prescribe in detail a remedy for this problem. Yet eminent medical authorities are proposing biennial medical exams for male politicians. I think that voters and constitutional experts should carefully consider the following points to see what might be done.

First, is it fair to say that the privilege of holding a public office should be contingent upon the man's maintaining the physical, mental, and emotional ability to discharge its duties with a reasonable degree of efficiency?

Second, should there be, for public men in the susceptible age bracket, a periodic review of physical and mental health and of conduct in office to see whether they are suffering from the male climacteric? Regular examinations, although not for this precise purpose, are imposed on airline pilots as a means of ensuring the safety of the traveling public.

Third, for those men who are found to be experiencing climacteric symptoms, should there be a compulsory course of treatment?

Finally, if any such men refuse to accept treatment, or fail to respond to it, should they be removed from office?

Glossary

Some of these words have various shades of meaning in popular usage. The meanings given here are the ones used in this book.

Allergy   Oversensitivity to certain substances (allergens) that are harmless to most people.

Androgens   Hormones that produce man's primary and secondary sex characteristics.

Androsterone   One of the male sex hormones.

Angina pectoris   A severe pain in chest, neck, or left arm, caused by a shortage of oxygen in the heart muscle.

Antidepressant   A drug that lifts the patient's mood and eases depressed feelings.

Antihedonistic   Opposed to pleasure seeking; puritanical.

Aphrodisiac   A drug or other remedy that arouses sexual desire.

Arteriosclerosis   Hardening of the arteries.

Atopic reaction   Allergic reaction at one point to an allergen applied elsewhere on the body.

Autonomic nervous system   Automatically regulates body functions not normally under conscious control; has two branches—the sympathetic and the parasympathetic.

Biopsy   Removal of live body cells for microscopic examination.

Birth control   Physical, chemical, hormonal, or other methods of preventing conception or birth.

Bisexual   Attracted to both sexes; also, having both male and female sexual organs (hermaphroditic).

Brain cortex   Outer layer of the brain hemispheres—"gray matter," the seat of consciousness.

Castration   Desexing of the male by removal of the testicles.

Climacteric   A major change, a turning point in human life.

Coitus   Sexual intercourse.

Conception   Fertilization, the joining of the male sperm with the female egg (ovum).

Contraception   See Birth control.

Corpus luteum Latin for "yellow body"; part of the ovary that produces the female hormone progesterone.

Depression An abnormal, long-lasting feeling of dejection; low spirits; "the blues."

Detuminescence See Resolution.

Diencephalon The midbrain; a structure connecting the hindbrain to the two cerebral hemispheres that make up the forebrain.

Dualism The doctrine that man consists of two separate parts—body and soul.

Endocrine glands Glands that secrete hormones directly into the bloodstream without a duct.

Endogenous Arising from causes within a person—for example, constitutional or genetic causes.

Erection Hardening and stiffness of the penis for sexual activity.

Erogenous zones Parts of the body susceptible to sexual stimulation —for example, neck, breasts, abdomen, and thighs.

Erotic Pertaining to or arousing sexual excitement.

Estrogens Ovarian hormones that produce woman's primary and secondary sex characteristics.

Exogenous Arising from causes outside a person in the environment —for example, other people's behavior or natural calamities.

Fertility In men the ability to produce live sperm; in women the ability to produce live ova.

Formication A tickling or stinging sensation like insects crawling on or under the skin.

Frigidity Absence of libido in women; reluctance to engage in sexual activity.

FSH Follicle stimulating hormone; in men it stimulates production of sperm.

Genitals The external sex organs.

Genitourinary system A group of organs concerned with reproduction and with production of urine. In men it includes kidneys, bladder, testicles, and penis; in women it includes kidneys, bladder, ovaries, womb and vagina.

Glands Organs that produce useful biochemical substances and release them into the system (for example, the pituitary) or that remove undesirable substances from the system (for example, the kidneys).

Gonadotrophins Pituitary hormones that stimulate the sex glands.

Gynecomastia   Enlarged breasts of a man, resembling those of a woman.

Hallucination   Sensory perception (visions or voices, for example) without any external origin, formed within the mind of the person.

Hedonistic   Motivated largely or entirely by a desire for pleasure.

Heterosexual   Attracted to the other sex.

Homosexual   Attracted to the same sex.

Hormone   A chemical messenger produced by a ductless gland and carried by the blood to another part of the body, which it stimulates to action.

Hypothalamus   A region of the brain that links the central and autonomic nervous systems; controls the glands.

ICSH   Interstitial cell stimulating hormone; same as LH, the luteinizing hormone.

Illusion   A false interpretation of a real sensory perception; a misconception of reality.

Impotence   Inability in men to have an erection of the penis sufficient for sexual intercourse.

Infertility   Inability of men to produce sperm or of women to produce ova adequate for reproduction.

Interstitial cells   A part of the testicles that produces male hormones, including testosterone.

LH   Luteinizing hormone; in men it stimulates production of male hormones, including testosterone; another name for ICSH.

Libido   Desire for sexual activity.

Meninges   Membranes between the inner surface of the skull and the brain.

Menopause   The time when a woman stops menstruating.

Metabolic   Pertaining to the chemical changes by which living tissue is built up or broken down.

Myalgia   A pain originating in a muscle.

Nervi erigentes   Nerve junctions in the pelvis; injury to them may cause impotence.

Neuralgia   A pain originating in a nerve.

Oedipus complex   Sexual attraction experienced by a son toward his mother; associated with father rivalry.

Osteoporosis Excessive porosity of the bones, with resulting reduction of hardness.

Ovaries Female glands producing sex hormones or eggs (ova).

Ovum The egg or female seed (plural, ova).

Parasympathetic nervous system A division of the autonomic nervous system; among its functions are focusing the eyes, slowing the heart, and stimulating the digestive system.

Paroxysmal tachycardia Excessively rapid beating of the heart without physical cause.

Peptic ulcer An open sore in the mucous membrane lining the esophagus, stomach, or duodenum.

Phallic Pertaining to the phallus, or penis.

Pituitary gland An important ductless gland located beneath the brain; its frontal part produces several important hormones, including the gonadotrophins LH and FSH.

Potency Ability to sustain erection of the penis for satisfying intercourse.

Prostate gland An organ surrounding the outlet of the bladder that produces the seminal fluid.

Pseudoangina A pain similar to angina pectoris, but not caused by a shortage of oxygen in the heart muscle; usually caused by chronic anxiety.

Psychosis A severe mental derangement; the person loses touch with reality.

Psychosomatic Referring to the mind-body interrelationship.

Repression Pushing unpleasant emotions into the unconscious part of the mind.

Resolution The loss of penile erection and subsidence of sexual excitement that follow orgasm in man; detuminescence.

Respiratory alkalosis Abnormal alkaline condition of the blood caused by overbreathing.

Semen A mixture of sperm with fluid from the prostate gland and seminal pouches (vesicles).

Sperm The male seed.

Sphincter A ring of muscle controlling the outlet of the bladder or anus.

Sterile Unable to produce seed.

Sterilization An operation to make a person sterile: in men by severing the spermatic cords and in women by severing the female egg tubes.

Sympathetic nervous system   A division of the autonomic nervous system; among its functions are stimulating sweat glands, speeding the heart, and suppressing digestive activity.

Syndrome   A group of symptoms characteristic of one disease or condition.

Testicles   Male sex glands in the scrotum.

Testosterone   The most important of the androgens, or male hormones.

Tetany   Muscular spasm of face, body, and limbs, resembling that produced by lockjaw.

Urethra   A tube that conveys urine from the bladder through the prostate gland and penis.

Urologist   Physician specializing in treatment of the genitourinary system.

Uterus   The womb; the hollow internal female organ for the growth of the embryo.

Vagina   The female sexual canal leading to the uterus.

Vasomotor nerves   Nerves that dilate (widen) or constrict (narrow) the blood vessels.

Virility   Potency plus fertility.

Index